Contents

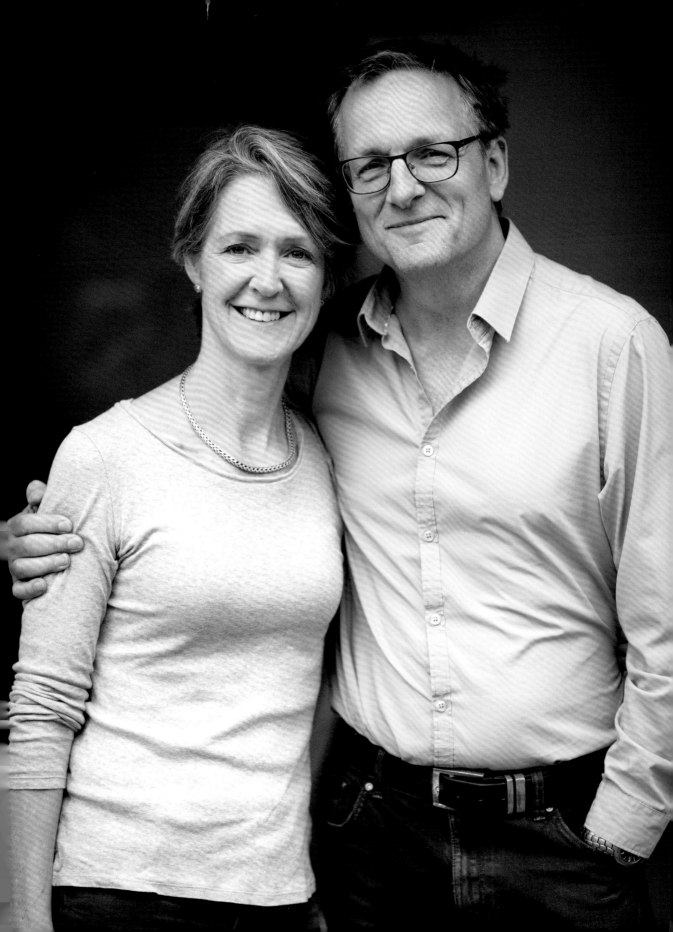

the fast
800
keto
recipe book

Foreword by Michael Mosley

Clare and I have written a number of books together in the ten years or so since I first discovered that I had type 2 diabetes and managed to reverse it by losing 9kg on an intermittent fasting diet, which I called my 5:2 plan. As the science on dietary health has evolved, so has our approach. Our most recent book, *The Fast 800 Keto*, incorporates the health-giving principles of combining a low-carb, keto Mediterranean diet with intermittent fasting – by which I mean eating 800–900 calories on a 'fast' day.

The 'keto' element acts as a turbo charger to intermittent fasting. There's compelling research to show that cutting back on sugars and starchy carbohydrates and increasing consumption of protein, such as meat, fish, tofu and eggs, allows your body to 'flip the metabolic switch' – to go from burning sugar to burning fat as your main fuel source. Your body does this by converting stored fat to ketone bodies, which is why a very low-carbohydrate diet is also known as a keto diet. Combining it with 800–900-calorie days helps you achieve ketosis. And going into ketosis not only leads to rapid weight loss, it promotes the release of the hunger-suppressing hormone ghrelin, so you don't feel hungry all the time.

One thing that often surprises people, when they ask me about a keto diet, is that it has been used for more than 100 years to treat epilepsy. Scientists have found that, as the brain increasingly relies on ketones for fuel, this reduces brain cell 'excitability' and therefore seizures. Which could explain why going into ketosis also helps mood. And there is mounting evidence that it can also help people with type 2 diabetes return their blood sugars to normal, without medication.

An important thing to be aware of is that there are different ways of going into ketosis, and we strongly recommend that you always opt for healthy sources of fat, carbs and protein (what I call a Med-style keto diet), as that ensures you get plenty of all the right nutrients, while cutting back on the junk.

When Clare and I used this approach to help a group of six unhealthy volunteers for a Channel 4 television series, 'Lose a Stone in 21 Days', they were really impressed with how easy they found it. Once they had gone into ketosis they weren't tormented by hunger pangs and they not only lost significant amounts of weight – fast – but also saw big improvements in their blood sugar levels, blood pressure, mood and overall energy.

I'm pleased to say they are still doing well. And that's because research has also shown that this approach is effective at keeping the weight off. So, whether you want to lose weight fast, harness the many health benefits of intermittent fasting, or just slow the encroachment of middle-age spread, the Fast 800 Keto plan provides a highly nutritious and extremely adaptable way of eating.

The big question is what are you going to eat and drink while on this diet? That's where Clare's latest recipes come in. They are simple to prepare, delicious and carefully balanced to ensure that you get all the necessary nutrients. I've thoroughly enjoyed being her chief taster – and I'm sure you'll love the recipes, too!

Fast, Easy, No-nonsense Keto

When Michael and I met at medical school, back in the early 1980s, what we learned about nutrition could have been scribbled on the back of an envelope. The basic message was 'eat less, move more' and, until a few years ago, like most doctors, I gave out this standard diet advice – then watched in alarm as my patients continued to put on weight and get sicker.

The trouble with the 'eat less, move more' approach to weight loss is that it ignores the impact that different foods have on our appetites and assumes that all calories are pretty much the same. As we now know, different foods are digested in different ways and have different effects on our bodies and brains, as well as our hunger levels. Proteins and fats, for example, have little impact on our blood sugar levels, while eating lots of sugary carbs will make them soar, increase food cravings and help pile on the fat. This, in turn, can lead to high blood pressure, raised blood fats, pre-diabetes and even full-blown type 2 diabetes.

As for 'moving more', lots of studies have shown that, on its own, increasing your activity level is not an easy way to lose weight. Doing exercise doesn't burn anything like as many calories as you might think, and it can also make you hungrier. Being active is good for your wellbeing, but not necessarily for your waistline.

Fortunately, there has been a sea change in our understanding of how to lose weight sustainably in the last decade – one that Michael has helped pioneer. When he embarked on his journey of discovery with the 5:2 diet, back in 2012, I watched at first with some scepticism, and then with great interest. Instead of 'eat less, move more', his programme involved starting with rapid weight loss via intermittent fasting – based on a lowish-carb Mediterranean-style diet. Here, finally, was an approach that made good scientific sense.

I soon found myself recommending Michael's diet plans to patients. And at home, too, I have thoroughly enjoyed our gradual switch to a lowish-carb Mediterranean-style diet. To be honest, that is how I have always enjoyed eating, but with four children, chicken and chips had taken over! So, it has been an incredibly satisfying experience, finding ways to get back to eating real food, improving our protein intake and reducing our consumption of starchy carbohydrates and sugar, as the science of nutrition has evolved.

These days, Michael and I work as a team: he researches the latest science, talks to leading scientists and finds clever ways to present his findings to huge audiences around the world; I also get involved in scientific studies (more on this below), while indulging my love of cooking, through creating and adapting recipes to support the Fast 800 plan.

I hope you will find plenty to choose from in this new book, which provides lots of tasty, nutritious meals that are easy to prepare and, crucially, use readily available and affordable ingredients.

In the past, ketogenic diets tended to be very high in fat and low in fibre, and involve a lot of meat eating, making them hard to sustain. Our low-calorie Mediterranean keto diet is simpler, cheaper and healthier; it is also better for the environment. The great thing about it is the combination of eating a healthy keto-style diet *and* restricting your calorie intake. This makes it easier to go into ketosis, helps reduce your appetite, accelerate weight loss and preserve your muscle mass. And, when it comes to carbs, it isn't as restrictive as other ketogenic regimes. As it is based on the Mediterranean diet, you can still eat some whole grains, beans, lentils, fruits and other occasional treats (indeed, for those of you who, like Michael, love their puddings, we have created some scrumptious low-carb desserts, cakes and biscuits that will not put your diet at risk).

Countless patients and readers have told me that they are surprised they no longer feel hungry on this diet – and that they have more energy and mental clarity, too. As for losing weight and keeping it off, this has been demonstrated in a number of clinical trials, including one I helped set up, the DIAMOND Study, which was led by Professor Susan Jebb from Oxford University. Published in 2019, this was the first randomised, controlled trial based on asking patients with obesity and type 2 diabetes to either eat a low-carbohydrate, real-food diet of 800–1000 calories a day (similar to the Fast 800 approach) or follow standard health advice. The results were impressive; the patients on the diet found it easy to stick to and not only lost an average of 9.5kg over three months, but also saw big improvements in their blood sugar levels, compared to the control group, despite having stopped some diabetes medications.

More recently, the Fast 800 Online Program has been independently validated by the Academic Health Sciences Network, part of the NHS's Office for Life Sciences. When they looked at data collected from thefast800.com participants, they found that those with obesity lost an average of 7.3kg in three months, rising to 8.7kg at 12 months; more than half of people with type 2 diabetes reduced their blood sugar levels to such an extent that by the end of three months their blood sugars were no longer in the diabetic range, despite many reducing medication; and nearly two thirds of overweight patients with prediabetes managed to get their blood sugars back into the normal healthy range.

Whether you are doing this programme via the Fast 800 books or online, the results are truly remarkable – people not only lose weight, but keep it off. What's more, the wider health benefits are increasingly clear, including decreased risk of type 2 diabetes, stroke and some cancers; reduced blood pressure, pain and inflammation; and improved mobility, mental health, sleep and mood.

If you would like extra support with the programme, visit our website www.thefast800.com, where you will find all sorts of useful resources.

I hope these recipes inspire you to try new meals and to experiment with the Fast 800 Keto approach. You'll be amazed to discover just how delicious and satisfying healthy eating can be.

Go for it!

Clare

PS Do follow me on Instagram @drclarebailey for recipes and related health tips. I love to hear how you are getting on!

A Note from Kathryn Bruton

Clare and I have had the joy of spending countless hours planning, testing and tweaking the recipes for this book. We were clear from the start that each recipe needed to be delicious while easy-to-find ingredients. It was also imperative that each recipe contained sufficient protein and fibre, while keeping sweet and starchy carbohydrates to a minimum. At times, it became a little bit like assembling a jigsaw or conducting an orchestra, as we worked to get the right fit. Our aim was to create recipes that work as well in your home as they have in our test kitchen, dishes that you will want to cook again and again. And I'm confident we've got there with these!

A Flexible, Three-stage Programme

STAGE 1

Rapid weight loss

The Fast 800 Keto starts with a low-calorie, ketogenic diet to kick-start fat-burning. It involves sticking to around 800–900 calories a day, eating two big, or three smaller, meals. All the recipes in this book are designed to help you do this. They are moderately high in protein (to keep you feeling fuller for longer) and low in carbohydrates and calories. However, on days when you are feeling hungry, you can choose from a range of keto-friendly top-ups to take your daily quota up to 1000 calories. You can stay in Stage 1 for anything from three to 12 weeks, before easing into Stage 2.

STAGE 2

Intermittent fasting

During this stage, you will continue to lose weight steadily, but at a slower rate, as some of the calorie restrictions are eased. You just pick two, three or four days each week as fast days, when you stick to 800–900 calories and keep carbohydrates to a minimum (as on Stage 1), and for the rest of the week you follow a lowish-carb Mediterranean-style diet not counting calories.

Many people skip Stage 1 and go straight to Stage 2, often following a 3:4 pattern, whereby they fast on Monday to Thursday, and then enjoy three relaxed days with no calorie counting at the weekend, adding complex carbohydrates, such as wholegrain bread, pasta, beans or lentils, to their meals. And lots of people move on to a 5:2 pattern, only cutting their calories 2 days a week.

Although each recipe is calorie counted, we have included plenty of 'adaptions' – such as doubling portions and adding 2–3 tablespoons of brown rice or a slice of seeded wholegrain bread – for your 'non-fast days', and to make it easy for you to adjust the dishes to suit everyone in the family. This means you can enjoy delicious and nutritious meals at every stage of your weight loss journey.

STAGE 3

Maintenance

This is the long-term weight maintenance phase when you turn the core principles of this diet into a way of life. Stage 3 enables you to enjoy a healthy, Mediterranean-style diet with plenty of protein (aiming for around 1g of protein per kilogram of body weight) and some complex carbohydrates. You can continue using the recipes in this book, including any of the top-ups, upping your portion size on days when you feel particularly hungry and occasionally enjoying a glass of wine or slice of cake with no need to count calories, hurrah! If the weight starts to creep back on, just add in a few fast days to get back on track.

Exclusions and Cautions

Rapid weight loss does not suit everyone. If you have a significant underlying medical condition, for example type 2 diabetes, and are on insulin or other medication; if you have blood pressure, moderate or severe retinopathy, epilepsy, gallstones, or are pregnant or breast-feeding, please talk to your doctor before going on this diet. It is not suitable for teenagers, people with a history of an eating disorder or a psychiatric illness, or if you are unwell, underweight or doing endurance exercise. See more: www.thefast800.com/frequently-asked-questions/

Keto strips

After a few days on the Fast 800 Keto, your body should go into ketosis – this is when it has used up its immediately available glucose stores and starts to burn excess body fat as fuel. As this happens, fatty acids are released from your fat stores and converted into ketone bodies, which can be used for energy by most cells in the body and brain.

You can check if you are in ketosis by using keto strips. These thin strips of plastic (available online or at pharmacies) have an active agent on one end, which you dip into your urine stream. The agent changes colour if it detects ketones in your urine. It's VERY motivating to see the strip turning red and a surprisingly useful deterrent if you are tempted by a biscuit! However, be aware that your ketone measurement tends to drop over a matter of weeks, even though you may be in ketosis and losing weight.

Time restricted eating (TRE)

We are fans of time-restricted eating because the science suggests that you will be healthier (and will find weight loss easier) if you limit your eating window and extend your normal overnight fast. Try eating your last meal at least three hours before you go to bed, and then delaying breakfast until an hour or so after you wake up. You may find you are happy to skip breakfast altogether on some days.

Throughout every stage of the Fast 800 Keto plan, you can choose whether to have two or three meals a day. At the back of the book, you'll find a series of meal plans, offering you a choice. Try the different approaches and see what works best for you.

The 'Rule of 50'

Many of us don't get enough good-quality protein, which is vital for all body functions, including immunity, building muscle, tissues, hormones and the building blocks for brain cells, blood and more. Furthermore, recent research shows it can also help us feel fuller for longer (and stop sugar cravings and the urge to overeat). The important thing is to ensure that protein comprises at least 15–20 per cent of the calories you eat. On an 800–900-calorie day, this means eating at least 50g of protein. We have carefully calibrated our recipes to help you do this, and listed how much there is in each recipe. See also the list of protein top-ups on page 240 – no need to count the calories – which you can use to adapt salads or veg dishes to suit your own taste.

If you're going it alone and creating your own recipes and menu plan, try and follow the Rule of 50 – i.e. more than 50g of protein and less than 50g of carbohydrate per day. Just check the protein and carb content on the packaging of any given item, or look it up online (e.g. one chicken breast is 31g of protein per 100g). Don't feel too worried if you are slightly out on any given day.

Eating enough protein can be challenging for vegetarians, and even more so for vegans, who may need to use supplements or consider increasing their daily calorie intake to over 1000, as explained in the FAQs. Using protein-rich, meal-replacement shakes (see www.thefast800.com for options) can be helpful here.

When you move to intermittent fasting in Stage 2, you will be eating more calories on non-fasting days, and you can further boost your protein intake. By the time you are happily at your target weight and on the maintenance stage of the plan, you can – and should – ensure your protein is upped to around 70–80g per day for women and 90–100g for men.

It's All About Real Food

As you will see from the recipes in this book, the Fast 800 Keto is about as far from a faddy diet as you can get. Based on a low-carb, Mediterranean-style way of eating, it's about simple, good food, as far as possible cooked from scratch. Here's a quick recap of what you should be aiming to eat and what you should be avoiding.

What to avoid:

❶ Ultra-processed foods (UPF)

Although fats, carbs and sugar have in turn been blamed for the current obesity crisis, there is mounting evidence that the real problem is that people are eating far too much ultra-processed food – food produced in factories which is typically high in poor-quality fat, carbs, sugar and salt, making it extremely calorific and hard to resist.

The foods in this group include some pretty obvious candidates, such as shop-bought chicken nuggets, burgers, chips, pizzas, hotdogs, fizzy drinks and fruit juices. But it also includes most mass-produced breads, biscuits, cakes, buns, sweetened breakfast cereals, crisps, energy bars, margarine and just about anything that says 'instant'– i.e. instant noodles, soups, desserts etc.

Not only are ultra-processed foods full of the unhealthy stuff, they also tend to be low in fibre, so we go on eating them without feeling sated. Furthermore, given that eating fibre is essential for keeping your gut bacteria in good shape, a diet high in ultra-processed foods is going to damage your microbiome and lead to inflammation in the gut and in the rest of the body, too.

How can you spot an ultra-processed food? It will probably be heavily packaged and heavily promoted. Read the label. If there are five or more ingredients, and those ingredients include numbers or have names you don't recognise, the chances are it's ultra-processed. Move quickly on!

❷ Sugar and sweeteners

There are lots of modern-day foods which are packed with sugar. What matters, though, is not just how much there is, but *when* you eat it and *what* you eat with it. If you eat sugary treats on an empty stomach, you are likely to get a rapid sugar spike in the blood, followed by a sugar crash, leaving you craving more. If you eat the same amount of sugar straight after a healthy meal, however, the sugar will be absorbed more slowly with a lower spike, thanks to the fat, fibre and protein in that meal.

The rules is: try not to eat sugary carbs, unless they come with fibre. The natural sugars you find in fruit or dates have less of an impact on your blood sugar levels because of the fibre they contain. And this is why, as far as possible, we use fruit when we want to add a touch of sweetness to our recipes. We do occasionally include small amounts of natural honey or maple syrup, but these contain other healthy nutrients (which refined table sugar does not).

The simplest way to reduce sugar in your diet is to cook your food from scratch – that way you know exactly what has gone into it. The 'hidden' sugars in ready-made convenience foods can be very hard to spot. If the word 'sugar' does not appear in the ingredients list, look out for alternative names, such as maltose, dextrose, fructose, glucose and lactose. There are more than 60 different names for what is essentially sugar, which can add up to be the main ingredient!

Artificial sweeteners are another challenge. They are many times sweeter than sugar, and can increase your sugar cravings. Some also damage the good microbes in your gut microbiome. If you have to use a sweetener, your best bet is probably stevia, which is based on a South American plant. Hopefully, while on the Fast 800 Keto diet, you'll find your tastes change and you'll enjoy treats with far less sugar as your palate adapts.

And what to embrace:

❶ Healthy fats
A healthy, Mediterranean-style diet contains plenty of 'good' fats, such as olive oil, oily fish and nuts, all of which have been shown to lower your risk of stroke and heart disease. For oily fish, think SMASH: Salmon, Mackerel, Anchovies, Sardines and Herring.

When it comes to plant-based fats, olive oil is the healthiest one to use. And with all varieties – olive, rapeseed, sunflower – the least processed the better. If you can afford it, buy cold-pressed or virgin oils, as they are unrefined and retain more of their natural nutrients.

❷ Dairy
The latest research shows that, when it comes to dairy, full-fat is best. Full-fat products are less processed and do *not* lead to weight gain or type 2 diabetes. Full-fat Greek-style yoghurt, for example, doesn't usually contain the starchy thickeners and sugars or sweeteners that are often added to enhance low-fat products.

❸ Meat
Although we are trying to eat less meat in general these days, for health and environmental reasons, it is an excellent source of good-quality protein. Try to buy better-quality, grass-fed varieties, if you can.

❹ Non-starchy veg
When you are trying to lose weight or control your blood sugars, it is best to stick to non-starchy vegetables, i.e. those that are lower in carbs and hidden sugars, such as spinach, cabbage, kale, pak choi, courgettes, aubergines and broccoli. On the Fast 800 Keto, we encourage you to enjoy generous portions of these, ideally filling half your plate with steamed greens, salad or any of the other vegetables featured in this book. They are so low in calories and provide such vital, gut-friendly fibre that they can be eaten freely – even with a drizzle of olive oil or a dressing (see No-count Dressings on pages 236–9).

❺ Fruit
Fruit contains lots of health-promoting phytonutrients and fibre – you should aim for one or two portions a day. But most of the phytonutrients and fibre are in the skin, so eat your fruit whole, rather than in the form of juice. Try to go for berries and hard fruits, such as pears and apples which have a lower sugar content, rather than sweet tropical varieties, like melons or pineapple.

As with sugary carbs, fruit is best eaten either with a meal or straight after a meal, rather than as a snack, when it's more likely to cause a sugar spike and be stored as fat.

How to Get the Most Out of the Plan and Stay on Track

❶ **Before you start**, take a little time to stop and really think about why you want to lose weight. Write down in a notebook or on the fridge what you want to achieve, the changes you want to see, and the reasons why weight loss or improved health is important to you. This is a key motivational tool, and something you can check back on if you find your willpower is beginning to waver.

❷ **Reduce temptation**. Go through your kitchen cupboards, fridge and freezer and either give away or throw away all 'off message' foods. Processed foods, sugary treats and snacks will not enhance your health, and as long as they are not within reach, they cannot tempt you. For the duration of this diet plan, make a pact with yourself not to buy any unhealthy foods.

❸ **Stock up on the good stuff**. In the keto phase of the diet, you are going to be eating plenty of healthy protein (fish, meat, tofu etc.). You will also be allowed generous amounts of leafy green vegetables (spinach, kale, cabbage, cabbage, cauliflower, Brussels sprouts etc.) and salad basics (lettuce, rocket, endive, cucumber, tomatoes, pepper etc.) drizzled with olive oil or dressing. You will need some complex carbs (chickpeas, lentils, quinoa and so on) and nuts and seeds for the occasional top-up, and do stock up on eggs as they make a great protein-rich breakfast, as well as a satisfying low-carb, low-calorie snack.

❹ **Tell friends, family and work colleagues**. Share the information that you are on a mission to improve your health and ask them to support you by not offering you cakes or wine. In fact, encourage them to try these recipes with you!

❺ **Aim to be more active**, but don't suddenly start doing strenuous sessions in the gym. Even doing a triathlon, you aren't going to be able to burn off enough calories to make a big difference to your body shape. That said, there's plenty of research to show that regular activity is good for just about every aspect of your mental and physical health. So, use your new healthy approach to food as an incentive to boost your activity levels, too – get out for a brisk walk, try to use the stairs instead of the lift, or do a few squats when you're waiting for the kettle to boil.

❻ **Prioritise sleep**. After a night of poor sleep you're more likely to be tempted by cravings and hunger pangs, so take steps to improve the quality of the sleep you get, whether that means switching off the TV and going to bed a bit earlier, experimenting with an eye mask and ear plugs (particularly useful if you sleep with someone who snores!), or creating a relaxing bedtime ritual of soft music and a warm bath.

❼ **Plan your meals ahead**. Set aside time every Sunday evening to plan meals for the week ahead. This might mean picking out recipes and ensuring you've got the ingredients you need and taking into account days when you've got time to cook, and days when you're more likely to be hungry and rushed. Many of our recipes can be prepared in double batches and then frozen, or whipped up in minutes from the contents of a well-stocked store cupboard, so you should never find yourself staring at a takeaway menu and tempted to reach for the phone!

8 **Keep a food/mood journal**. Studies show that keeping track of everything that passes your lips can be extremely helpful when you're trying to lose weight.

9 **Weigh yourself regularly**, and keep track of your fast-reducing waist measurement and blood pressure – studies show people who keep a close eye on their weight are more successful at keeping it off.

10 **Avoid snacking and eating on the hoof**. Make a point of sitting down at a table for all your meals – eating slowly and focusing on (and enjoying!) every mouthful.

11 **Keep well hydrated**. This is especially important on a fasting day when you are taking in less liquid with food and losing fluid when you burn fat. As a result, it's easy to get dehydrated and end up feeling exhausted, weak, light-headed or headachy.

On a fasting day aim to drink an extra 1–1.5 litres of calorie-free fluids, mainly as water (and more if you are very active or the weather is hot). You should be drinking enough water so that you are producing a good volume of urine 5–6 times a day. Sipping fluids can also distract you from cravings and reduce hunger pangs between meals.

Keep a large jug of water in the fridge and put in slices of lemon or cucumber for flavour. Try to avoid drinks with sweeteners, as they can upset the good bugs in your gut.

Tips for using this book:

Calorie counts
These refer to one individual serving, unless otherwise stated. That said, please be aware that we include calorie counts as a rough guide only. There are significant variations in measurements between different counters and apps, so don't be too concerned by a few extra calories here or there.

Suggestions for non-fast days
We offer plenty of tips if you are on Stage 2 or have moved on to the maintenance stage and wish to adapt the recipes to make them more substantial. This might involve increasing the portion size, adding a few tablespoons of brown rice or lentils, an extra glug of olive oil, a slice of seeded bread or more vegetables.

Make the recipes suit you
These recipes are based on the Mediterranean way of eating, but can be adapted to fit different cuisines and tastes. Feel free to adjust the flavours by adding different herbs and spices – it will have minimal impact on calories. The tastier and more satisfying your food, the more likely you are to stick to this way of eating.

FAQs

Will I feel hungry all the time?

For the first few days you are likely to feel hungry, but most people find that this settles as their metabolism resets and they go into ketosis. This is when keto strips can be particularly helpful. Seeing them change colour is incredibly motivating and will help keep you going as you get underway.

How many meals can I eat a day?

Some people like to stick to three meals a day, while others find it easier to control their calories on two – try both and see what works best for you (see TRE on page 11). However, we don't recommend splitting your daily calories across more than three meals – you need to give your body time to go into fat-burning mode. Nor do we suggest one meal a day, particularly if it's close to bedtime, as your body is more likely to treat it as a feast and store more fat.

Can I do the plan with meal replacement shakes?

Eating real food is generally best, but if you have limited healthy food at hand or when you're out, then good-quality shakes are a great alternative. As well as convenience, they give you the protein and nutrients you need and leave you feeling satisfyingly full. Do choose carefully as many shakes are full of sugars and contain inadequate amounts of protein (see www.thefast800.com for suitable low-carb, Mediterranean formula options).

Does the plan work for vegetarians? And vegans?

There's absolutely no reason why you can't do the Fast 800 Keto if you're a pescatarian (no meat, only fish) or a vegetarian. In fact, we've included lots of lovely fish-based and vegetarian recipes in this book, plus a vegetarian meal planner to get you started. If you are vegan, you will have to be clever in your protein choices, as many 'fake meat' products come with hidden carbohydrates which would take you out of ketosis. Even wholesome vegetable sources of protein, such as legumes and pulses, have quite a high carbohydrate content. Focus on high-protein foods, such as tofu, tempeh, edamame beans and seitan. Adding a big spoonful of nutritional yeast to soups and sauces can help, too. Because protein is so important, we suggest vegans allow themselves to go over 1000 calories, if necessary. (Do also make use of our protein top-ups on page 240 or try our low-carb protein powder or shakes at www. thefast800.com/meal-replacements/products/protein/.) You will still lose weight, just not quite as fast, and you may not go into ketosis. But that is OK.

Can I exercise on a fasting day?

If you are already doing exercise and feel comfortable sticking with it on a fasting day, carry on with your current regime. But don't start a new, heavy programme or do endurance exercise on a fasting day. A brisk walk is always a good idea, whatever your level of fitness.

Should I tell my health professional that I'm doing the diet?

It is always sensible to keep your health professional informed about a major change to your diet, particularly if you have a medical condition and/or are on medication. See Exclusions and Cautions on page 10.

Can I use the plan to target weight loss from certain parts of my body?

You can't 'target' specific areas, but studies show the Fast 800 approach is particularly good at rapidly reducing the fat that is stored in and around your middle (which tends to be the dangerous fat associated with other metabolic diseases, such as type 2 diabetes, heart disease and blood pressure) and around the neck.

If you are a woman and slim on top and around the middle, but have a build-up of fat on your bottom, thighs or upper arms which you struggle to lose (i.e. which is 'diet resistant'), then you may have lipoedema, which is the result of genetics and hormones. For more information, consult the Lipoedema Foundation or Lipoedema UK.

Should I take a multivitamin?

Our recipes are carefully balanced to include all the nutrients you need, but on a low-calorie diet it is not always easy to combine your meals for maximum nutritional variety, so we recommend taking a good-quality multivitamin on your 800-calorie days as a backup.

Can I have a drink?

It's best to cut out alcohol completely during Stage 1 and to just have the odd drink at weekends during Stage 2. Alcohol is extremely calorific – a single glass of wine can contain between 200 and 300 calories and ends up stored in the liver as fat, causing inflammation. It also weakens your willpower, so you're better off without it!

Will I experience any side effects?

There are four main side effects. People sometimes experience 'keto flu' as the body adapts to a different fuel. If you have been burning mainly sugar, your switch to burning fat can leave you feeling off-colour for a few days. This should soon pass and most people find that when they go into ketosis they feel better. However, it doesn't suit everyone.

If your symptoms are severe or don't settle over a few days, it would be a good idea to discuss this with your health professional before you continue. See the www.thefast800.com for more information.

Dehydration is probably the most common side effect, causing headaches, constipation and fatigue. It is important to make sure you are getting plenty to drink on an 800–900 calorie day. You are likely to be well hydrated if your urine is the colour of lemonade and you are passing a good volume about 5–6 times a day. (For more on keeping hydrated see page 15.)

Within days of embarking on a low-calorie keto diet, you may see your blood pressure drop – which can be a benefit, if it has been raised. But if you are on medication, particularly for raised blood pressure, or have any other medical condition, it is important to speak to your health professional before starting, as your medication may need monitoring and possibly to be reduced.

Constipation is a common side effect of being on a diet, particularly a keto diet, as fibre in the form of beans, pulses, wholegrains and many fruits is usually restricted. Because fibre is very important to a healthy gut – aiding weight loss and providing health benefits, such as improved immunity, reduced inflammation and even improving mood – we include healthy complex carbohydrates in moderation in our recipes.

Is it expensive?

We have done our best to ensure that the food in our recipes is practical and affordable. You will see that we encourage the use of jarred, tinned and frozen ingredients wherever possible, and we offer alternatives where suitable.

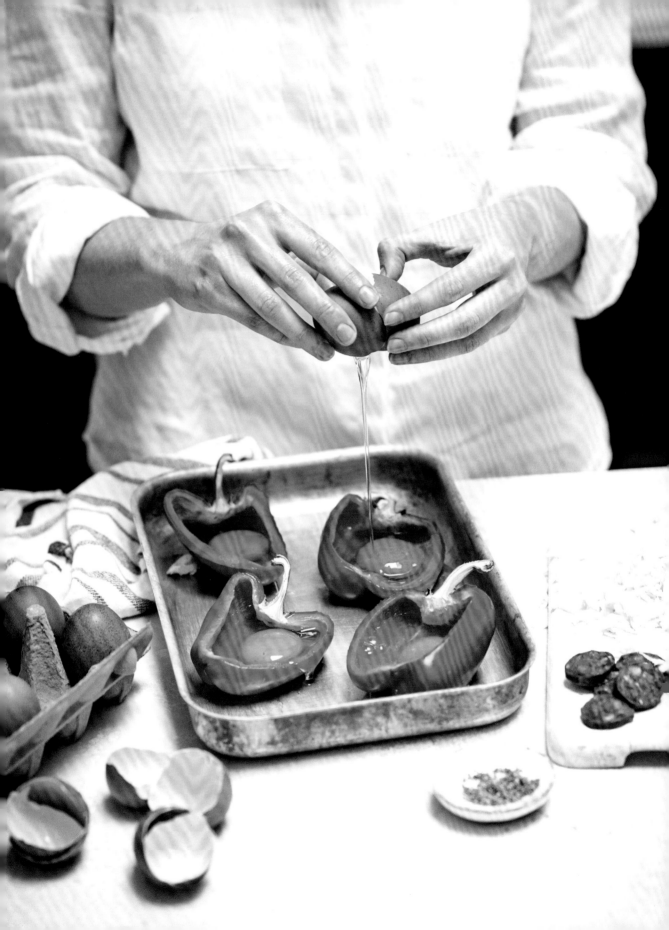

Breakfast & Brunch

For breakfast, think eggs, eggs and
more eggs. We love them. But don't
worry if they're not your thing; there
are plenty of other options here.
And, if you are someone who likes
to delay breaking their fast until
late morning or even lunchtime,
you might want to try some of the
more substantial brunch options -
Cauli-rice Kedgeree, anyone?

PER SERVING | **209cals** | PROTEIN **6.8g** | CARBS **18.1g**

Blueberry Bircher Muesli

SERVES **1** | PREP **5** mins

1 level tbsp oats
1 level tbsp chia seeds
1 heaped tbsp frozen
    blueberries
3 tbsp full-fat Greek yoghurt
    (approx. 45g)
1 tbsp full-fat milk
½ tsp ground cinnamon

NON-FAST DAY
Add a handful of chopped nuts
and/or serve a larger portion.

A nice little overnight muesli that can be easily thrown together using a tablespoon measure and some frozen blueberries. There is no need to defrost frozen blueberries prior to making this, as they will defrost in the fridge overnight. The chia seeds add protein, fibre and a creamy texture.

1. Place all the ingredients in a bowl, mix well and refrigerate overnight.

2. Stir to break up the blueberries before serving. Add an extra tablespoon of milk, if the mixture is too thick.

PER SERVING | **251cals** | PROTEIN **17.6g** | CARBS **22.9g**

Blueberry and Chocolate Protein Smoothie

SERVES **1** | PREP **3–4** mins

100g silken tofu
100g Greek yoghurt
50g frozen blueberries
1 medjool date, stone removed
1 tsp vanilla extract
1 tsp cocoa powder

This creamy smoothie gets a protein boost thanks to the tofu, while the cocoa not only adds flavour, it's also surprisingly high in fibre. Ideal for taking to work or for breakfast in a hurry.

1. Place all the ingredients in a blender and blitz until smooth.

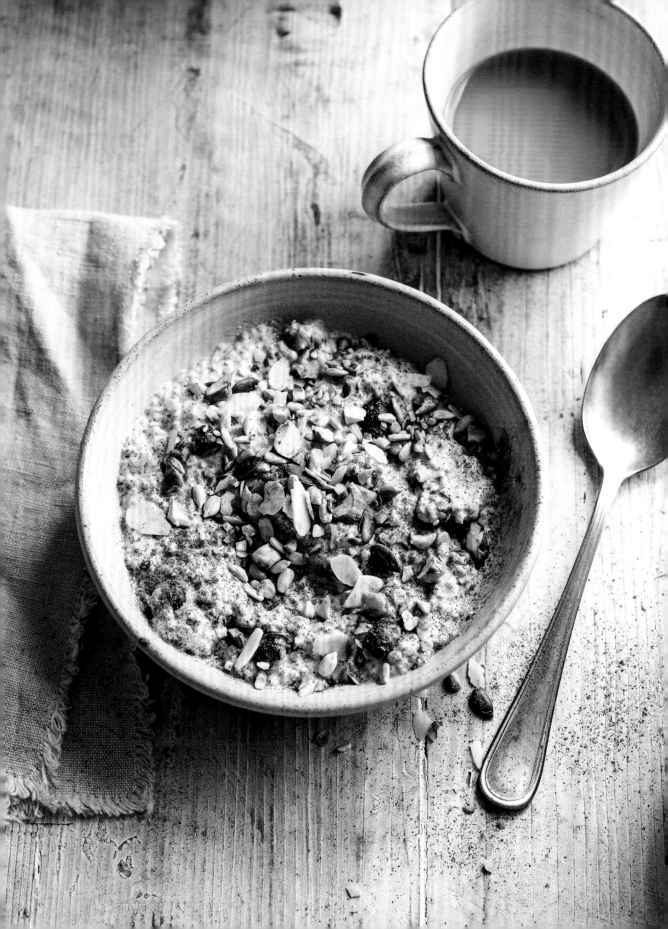

UNDER **200** CALORIES | PER SERVING | **105cals** | PROTEIN **3.7g** | CARBS **2.2g**

Keto Granola

SERVES	PREP	COOK
12	**5** mins	**5–7** mins

50g pumpkin seeds
50g sunflower seeds
20g linseeds
40g flaked almonds
40g pecan nuts, broken
    into small pieces
1 tsp vanilla extract
1 tsp ground cinnamon
1 tsp maple syrup
Pinch of salt

A nutty and seedy keto granola – delicately flavoured, wonderfully crunchy and satisfying. A little goes a long way.

1. Preheat the oven to 200°C/Fan 180°C/Gas 6.

2. Place all the ingredients in a bowl and mix well to combine.

3. Tip on to a baking tray and bake in the oven for 5–7 minutes, or until golden and crisp.

4. Allow to cool before serving. Store in an airtight container or jar.

UNDER **300** CALORIES | PER SERVING | **232cals** | PROTEIN **10.8g** | CARBS **7.1g**

Keto Granola Breakfast Bowl

SERVES	PREP	COOK
1	**2** mins	**0** mins

3 tbsp full-fat Greek yoghurt
2 tbsp Keto Granola
    (see above)
30g mixed berries
    (e.g. strawberries,
    raspberries, blueberries)

NON-FAST DAY
Increase the portion size, add extra nuts and half an unpeeled apple or pear, diced or grated.

Enjoy the granola crunch with creamy yoghurt and berries.

1. Combine all the ingredients in a bowl and serve.

Smashed Avocado on Fried Halloumi with Tomatoes and Egg

SERVES | PREP | COOK
1 | **5** mins | **3–4** mins

½ small, soft and ripe avocado
½ tsp fresh lemon juice
Pinch of chilli flakes
1½ tsp olive oil
65g halloumi, cut
    lengthways into 2
3 cherry tomatoes, quartered
1 medium egg

COOK'S TIP
Frying the egg for 3 minutes will give a runny yolk. Cook for a little longer, if you prefer.

NON-FAST DAY
Double the portion size.

Smashed avocado on toast is such a favourite for brunch. Here the fried halloumi takes the place of starchy bread, to make a firm and tasty base. Serve a colourful, leafy salad alongside.

1. Place the avocado flesh in a bowl with the lemon juice, chilli flakes, ½ teaspoon of the olive oil and some salt and freshly ground black pepper. Mash with a fork until combined but still slightly chunky.

2. Place the remaining oil in a frying pan over a medium heat. Add the halloumi slices, quartered tomatoes and crack in the egg. Fry everything for 3 minutes, turning the halloumi halfway through.

3. When the egg is cooked and the halloumi nicely browned, transfer the halloumi to a plate. Spread the smashed avocado over the cheese, top with the tomatoes and egg, and serve.

Harissa Yoghurt with Soft-boiled Eggs and Spinach

SERVES	PREP	COOK
1	**2** mins	**6** mins

2 medium free-range eggs
100g fresh spinach
2 tbsp Greek yoghurt
1 tbsp rose harissa pesto
    or ½ tbsp harissa paste
a few chilli flakes (optional)
1 tsp mixed seeds, toasted

COOK'S TIP

If you prefer less heat, substitute sun-dried tomato pesto for the harissa.

NON-FAST DAY

Serve with a thin slice of wholemeal bread, sourdough, or 2–3 tablespoons of quinoa.

A quick, easy breakfast with North African flavours. The creamy yoghurt adds extra protein and a tangy contrast to the crunchy seeds.

1. Bring a small pot of water to the boil and carefully lower in the eggs. Simmer for 5½ minutes. Using a slotted spoon, transfer the eggs to a bowl of iced water. Carefully peel the eggs and slice each one in half.

2. Remove the pan from the heat and plunge the spinach into the hot water. Stir for 30 seconds, then drain thoroughly and squeeze as much liquid as possible from the spinach.

3. Meanwhile mix the yoghurt and harissa together in a wide bowl.

4. Mix the drained spinach into the yoghurt. Season generously with salt and freshly ground black pepper, then top with the eggs, chilli flakes, if using, and a sprinkling of mixed seeds.

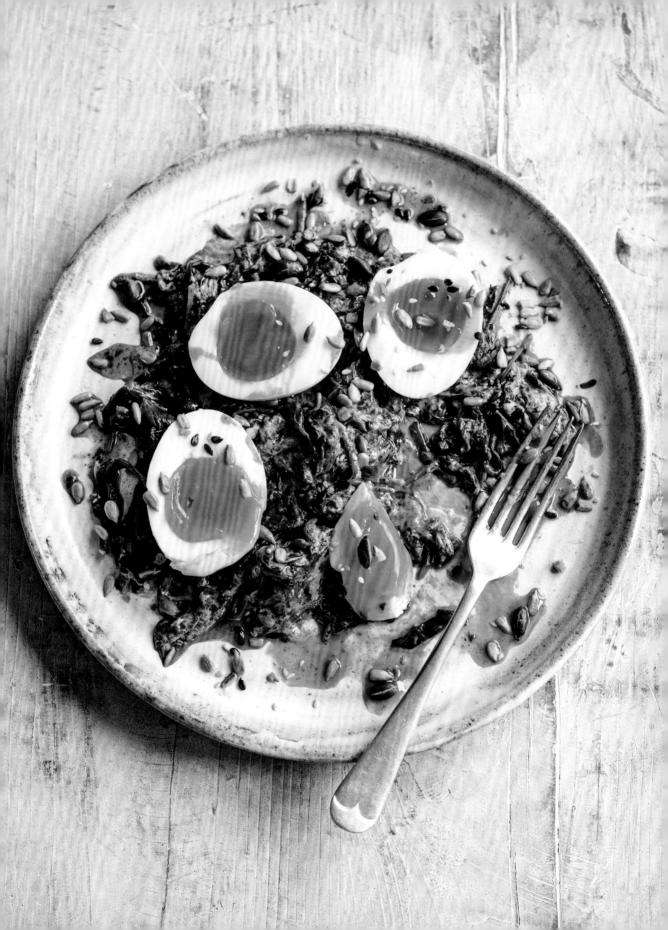

PER SERVING | **276cals** | PROTEIN **21.8g** | CARBS **6.2g**

Veg and Egg Breakfast Bake

SERVES	PREP	COOK
2	**10** mins	**15** mins

2 small red or yellow peppers,
   deseeded and finely chopped
2 spring onions, finely chopped
80g fresh spinach, roughly
   chopped
4 medium free-range eggs
1 tsp harissa (optional)
60g ricotta
40g feta cheese

NON-FAST DAY
Add a few unpeeled, cooked
baby potatoes to the egg
mixture before baking, or
serve with 2–3 tablespoons
wholegrain rice, quinoa
or bulgur wheat alongside
for lunch.

This remarkably versatile dish works well for breakfast,
lunch or supper. It can be served hot or cold, and can be
eaten at home or on the go and will keep for a couple of
days in the fridge. Serve with a light salad, if you like.

1. Preheat the oven to 200°C/Fan 180°C/Gas 6 and line
a 20cm square baking dish with baking parchment.

2. Place the peppers, spring onions and spinach in
a heatproof bowl, add 1 tablespoon water, cover and
microwave for 3 minutes. Tip into a sieve to drain
off any liquid.

3. Whisk the eggs, harissa, if using, and ricotta in a bowl
until thoroughly combined. Season generously with salt
and freshly ground black pepper.

4. Add the steamed veg to the egg mixture, stir well to
combine and transfer to the prepared dish. Crumble
the feta cheese over the top and bake in the oven for
15 minutes, or until set.

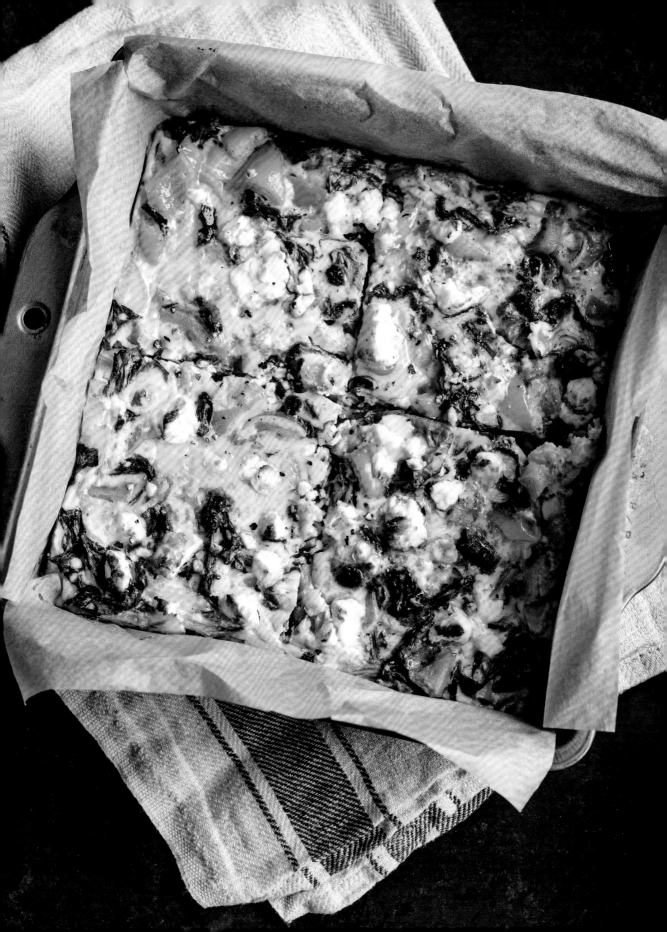

Fried Egg Makeover

These are fast food recipes, ready in minutes, using store cupboard ingredients and fridge staples to supercharge your morning eggs.

UNDER 200 CALORIES | PER SERVING | **195cals** | PROTEIN **16.8g** | CARBS **1.4g**

Mushroom and Miso Eggs with Spinach

SERVES	PREP	COOK
1	2 mins	5 mins

1 large Portobello mushroom, finely sliced
1 tsp olive oil
1 tsp white miso paste
20g fresh spinach, roughly chopped
2 medium free-range eggs

NON-FAST DAYS
Place the egg on a slice of seeded sourdough or wholemeal bread and add some salad, if you like.

Here the miso paste brings an exotic umami flavour to the mushrooms and spinach. Miso is quite salty so some freshly ground black pepper should suffice for seasoning.

1. Place the mushroom and oil in a frying pan over a medium heat and fry for 2 minutes until soft.

2. Mix the miso with ½ teaspoon boiling water to loosen, then stir into the mushrooms. Follow with the spinach and stir until wilted.

3. Crack the eggs on top of the vegetables, season with freshly ground black pepper, cover with a lid or baking tray and cook for 2 minutes, or until the eggs are set.

4. Serve immediately.

Black Olive and Toasted Almond Eggs

SERVES | PREP | COOK
1 | **2** mins | **2½** mins

35g pitted black olives,
    finely chopped
1 tsp olive oil
2 medium free-range eggs
1 heaped tbsp flaked
    almonds, toasted

Enjoy Mediterranean flavours for breakfast.
Kalamata olives have the best flavour, in my opinion,
but any olives would work well.

1. Place the olives and oil in a small frying pan over a
medium heat. Cook for 30 seconds, then crack the eggs
on top. Season with salt and freshly ground black pepper,
scatter the almonds all over, cover with a lid or baking
tray and cook for 2 minutes, or until the eggs are just set.

2. Serve immediately.

PER SERVING | **324cals** | PROTEIN **22.3g** | CARBS **5.9g**

Roasted Pepper and Halloumi Eggs

SERVES | PREP | COOK
1 | **3–4** mins | **5** mins

1 roasted red pepper from a jar,
    finely chopped (approx. 85g)
40g halloumi, finely diced
1 tsp olive oil
2 medium free-range eggs

This breakfast will bring a bit of colour and sunshine
to your morning.

1. Place the peppers, halloumi and oil in a frying pan
over a medium heat. Cook for about 2½ minutes,
until the halloumi is golden.

2. Crack the eggs into the pan and season with salt and
freshly ground black pepper. Cover with a lid or baking
tray and cook for 2 more minutes, or until the eggs are set.

3. Serve immediately.

PER SERVING | **365cals** | PROTEIN **16.1g** | CARBS **9.8g**

Cottage Cheese Crepes with Bacon, Avocado and Oven-roasted Tomatoes

SERVES	PREP	COOK
2	**10** mins	**10–12** mins

4 rashers smoked
   streaky bacon
8 cherry tomatoes, halved
1 small avocado, peeled,
   stoned and sliced
Juice of ½ lime
70g full-fat cottage cheese
1 medium egg
1 tbsp stoneground,
   wholemeal or
   buckwheat flour
small knob of butter,
   for frying

NON-FAST DAY
Add an egg, cooked
however you like it.

A keto twist on a traditional crepe, served with crispy bacon, oven-roasted tomatoes and avocado. My grown-up children love this. If you're serving it for lunch, you could add a handful of baby leaves and a no-count dressing (see pages 236–9).

1. Preheat the oven to 200°C/Fan 180°C/Gas 6 and line a baking tray with baking parchment.

2. Place the bacon and tomatoes on the prepared baking tray and roast in the oven for 10 minutes, or until the bacon is crispy and the tomatoes are bursting and juicy.

3. Dress the avocado slices with the lime juice, season with salt and freshly ground black pepper and set aside.

4. Measure 40g of the cottage cheese, the egg and flour into a bowl or jug and use a stick blender to blitz until smooth. Season well.

5. Place a non-stick frying pan over a medium heat and melt a small knob of butter. Pour in half the batter and tilt the pan so that it spreads out in a thin circle. Leave to cook for 1½–2 minutes. It is important to make sure it is fully cooked underneath in order to flip it easily. Carefully turn the crepe over, then cook for a further 30–40 seconds on the other side. Repeat with the remaining batter.

6. Spread half the remaining cottage cheese over one crepe and place 2 bacon slices and half the avocado and tomatoes on one side. Fold over to serve. Repeat with the remaining ingredients.

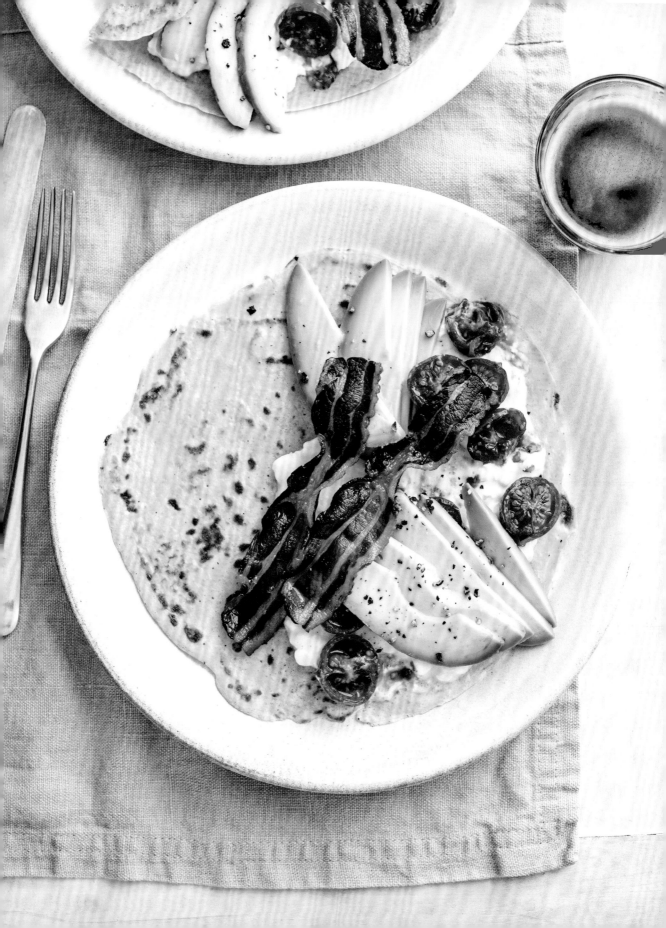

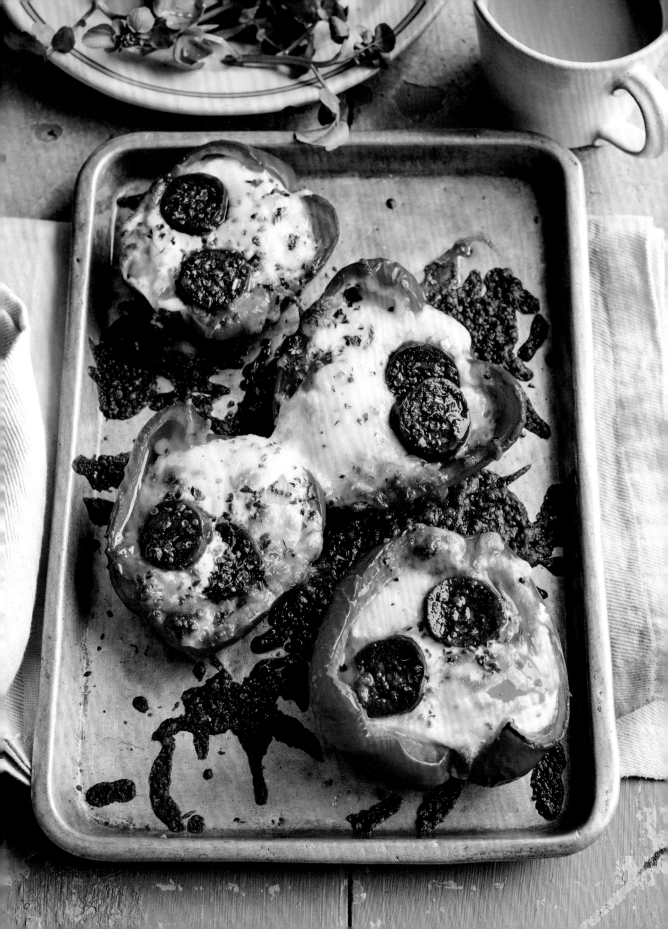

Baked Eggs in Peppers

SERVES	PREP	COOK
2	**5** mins	**20** mins

1 medium red pepper,
   halved and deseeded
2 medium free-range eggs
75g grated mozzarella
15g chorizo, sliced into 4
Pinch of dried oregano
   or thyme (optional)
½ tbsp olive oil, plus extra
   for greasing

COOK'S TIP

If you have calories to spare, or it's not an 800kcal day, you could mop the juices up with Instant Mug Bread (see page 206) or the Cloud Bread (see page 205).

NON-FAST DAY

Enjoy a double portion or serve with a slice of sourdough or wholemeal bread, or add 2–3 tablespoons of quinoa.

Red peppers are the perfect, juicy container for cooking eggs – here, they are enticingly flavoured with chorizo and melted mozzarella. For a more filling meal, serve on top of a large handful of bitter leaves, such as rocket, watercress or spinach.

1. Preheat the oven to 200°C/Fan 180°C/Gas 6 and lightly oil a baking tray.

2. Place the pepper halves cut-side-up on the prepared tray and roast in the oven for 5 minutes.

3. Carefully remove the pepper halves from the oven and crack an egg into each one. Top with the grated mozzarella, sliced chorizo, herbs, if using, and a drizzle of olive oil. Return to the oven for about 15 minutes, or until the cheese is bubbling and turning golden.

PER SERVING | **269cals** | PROTEIN **19.4g** | CARBS **2.8g**

Chorizo Omelette

SERVES	PREP	COOK
2	**5** mins	**5–7** mins

½ tbsp olive oil
½ small onion, peeled
    and finely diced
4 medium free-range eggs
3cm piece cured chorizo,
    sliced and quartered
30g Cheddar, grated
60g cooked or leftover greens
½ tsp chilli flakes (optional)

NON-FAST DAY
Have a larger portion.

This is one of Michael's go-to omelettes, which he cooks to perfection. It has fabulous Spanish flavours, is high in protein and is easy to make. It's even better topped with fermented veg, like sauerkraut, which adds a delicious sweet, salty and tangy flavour, and is so beneficial to your health that you don't need to count the calories.

1. Place a non-stick frying pan over a medium heat. Add the oil and onion and sweat for 2 minutes.

2. Crack the eggs into a small bowl and whisk with a fork. Season well with freshly ground black pepper, then pour over the onion. Leave for 30 seconds to start to set, then use a spatula or wooden spoon to pull the egg into the centre of the pan, allowing the runny mixture to flow out into the empty space. Do this 4 or 5 times, working quite quickly.

3. When the omelette has started to set, add the chorizo, cheese and greens. Cook for another 2 minutes, then scatter over the chilli flakes, if using. Fold one half of the omelette over the other and slide onto a plate to serve.

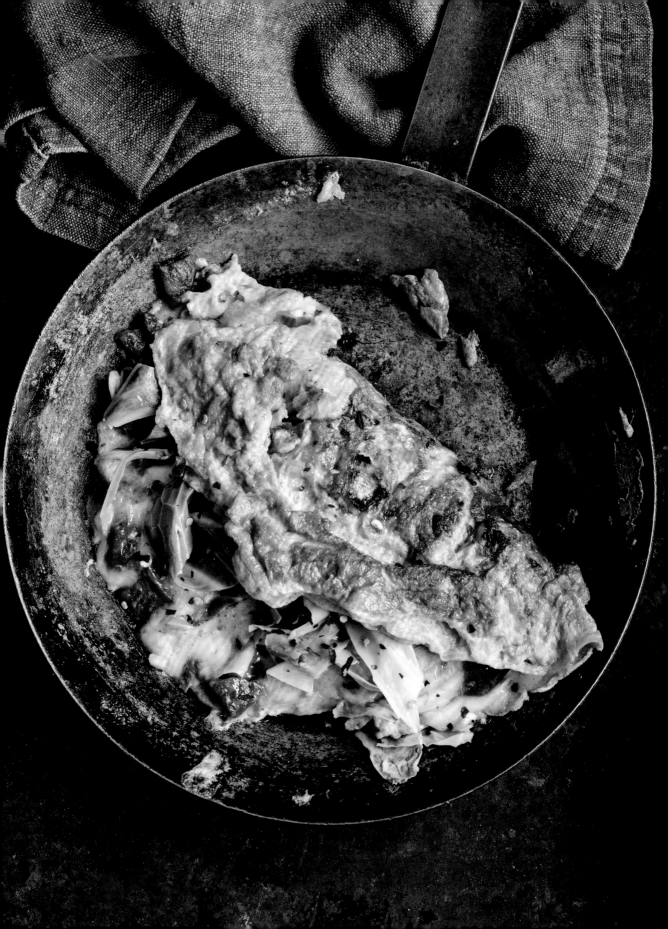

Basic Scrambled Eggs

SERVES	PREP	COOK
1	**1** mins	**3–4** mins

2 medium free-range eggs

COOK'S TIP
Fresh herbs, such as parsley or chives, would make a nice garnish.

NON-FAST DAY
Add a slice of seeded sourdough or wholegrain toast, or double the portion.

Eggs are a keto superfood – low in calories and carbs, and high in protein and nutrients. They have been re-evaluated since the days of low-fat diets, so it's OK to enjoy one or two eggs a day. We certainly do, as they leave you feeling full and less likely to reach for a snack. Here are three variations on the simple but ever-popular scrambled eggs. You can add rocket, baby spinach or cooked leafy greens to make any of these a more substantial meal, without having to count the extra calories.

1. Break the eggs into a small non-stick saucepan and whisk. (There is no need to do this in a separate bowl.)

2. Place over a very low heat and start stirring with a rubber spatula or wooden spoon. Keep stirring all the time until the eggs begin to cook. Thick silky lumps will begin to form as you stir. Carry on stirring until the eggs are cooked – they should still be loose and moist. Immediately remove from the heat as they will continue to cook.

Big Mushrooms with Anchovies and Scrambled Eggs

SERVES **1** | PREP **2–3** mins | COOK **15** mins

2 large mushrooms,
    stalks removed
2 anchovies in olive oil, diced
1 portion scrambled eggs
    (opposite)
20g rocket (optional)

These mushrooms are big on flavour and are filling, too. The anchovies give everything a lovely saltiness.

1. Preheat the oven to 200°C/Fan 180°C/Gas 6 and line a baking tray with baking parchment.

2. Place the mushrooms on the prepared tray and scatter the anchovies over them. Drizzle with 1 teaspoon of the anchovy oil and season with some freshly ground black pepper. Roast in the oven for 15 minutes.

3. Meanwhile, scramble the eggs as opposite.

4. When the mushrooms are ready, top with scrambled eggs and rocket, if using, to serve.

Greek Scrambled Eggs

SERVES **1** | PREP **2–3** mins | COOK **5–6** mins

1 medium tomato, coarsely
    grated and skin discarded
1 tbsp olive oil
Pinch of paprika (optional)
2 medium free-range eggs,
    whisked
15g feta cheese, crumbled
    (optional)

These eggs include extra protein and flavour, thanks to the feta, and a delicious, quick-to-make tomato paste.

1. Place the grated tomato in a non-stick frying pan with the olive oil and simmer over a medium heat for 3–4 minutes, stirring occasionally, until reduced to a thick paste. Stir in the paprika, if using.

2. Reduce the heat to low, pour in the eggs and stir. Gently scramble, stirring with a spatula all the time, for 1½ minutes.

3. Remove from the heat, season with salt and freshly ground black pepper and top with feta, if using, to serve.

Scrambled Eggs with Harissa Sautéed Kale and Soy Roasted Seeds

SERVES	PREP	COOK
1 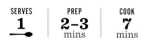	**2–3** mins	**7** mins

100g curly kale, sliced
1 tsp olive oil
½ tbsp harissa paste
2 tbsp full-fat Greek yoghurt
1 portion scrambled eggs
   (see page 36)
1 tbsp Soy Roasted Seeds
   (see page 194)

If you don't have the Soy Roasted Seeds from page 194 to hand, simply scatter 1 tablespoon pumpkin or sunflower seeds over the top and season with a sprinkle of salt. To enhance the flavour, toast the seeds first in a pan until golden.

1. Place the kale and olive oil in a medium pan with a lid, season with freshly ground black pepper and cook gently for 2–3 minutes, stirring once or twice.

2. Remove from the heat and stir in the harissa and yoghurt.

3. Cook the scrambled eggs as per instructions on page 36.

4. Serve the eggs with the kale and some Soy Roasted Seeds sprinkled over the top.

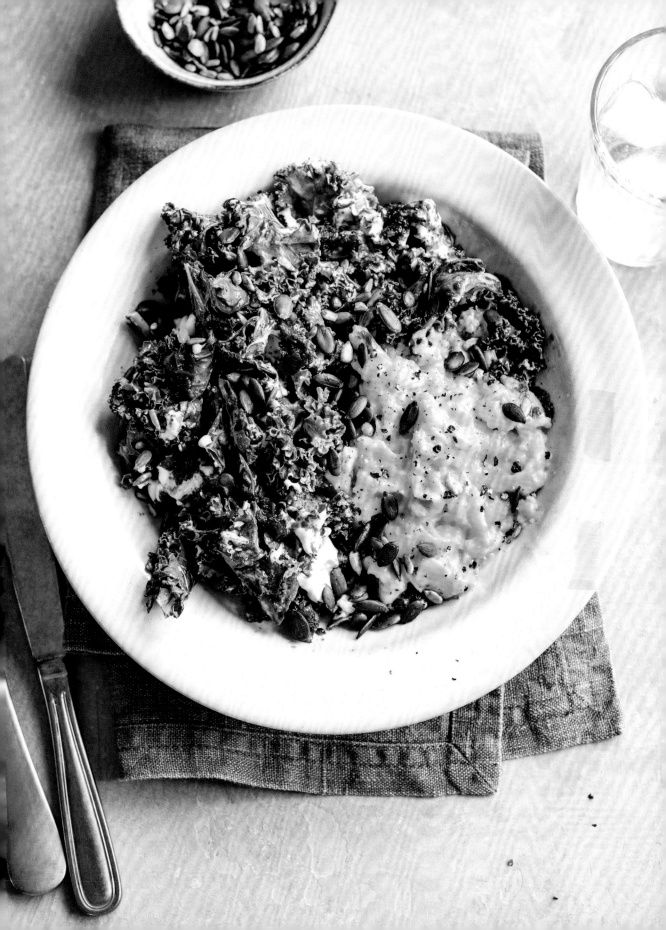

PER SERVING | **473cals** | PROTEIN **40.3g** | CARBS **27.4g**

Cauli-rice Kedgeree

SERVES **2** | PREP **20** mins | COOK **20** mins

2 medium free-range eggs
1 medium onion, peeled,
    ½ diced and ½ sliced
    into rings
1½ tbsp olive oil
1 tsp curry powder
2 bay leaves (optional)
2 skinless smoked haddock
    fillets (approx. 120g each)
200ml full-fat milk
25g raisins
¼ large cauliflower, grated
1 small courgette, finely sliced
1 tbsp chia seeds
Generous bunch flat-leaf
    parsley, roughly chopped
1 tsp fresh lemon juice

COOK'S TIP
If you can't find skinless
haddock fillets, simply
remove the skin before
cooking.

NON-FAST DAY
Scatter with toasted flaked
almonds and add a dollop
of butter while it is still hot.

You simply won't notice that the starchy rice has been replaced by nutritious, low-carb cauli-rice in this dish. It can be eaten hot or at room temperature. You could add steamed greens for a bit of colour and bite.

1. Place a small saucepan filled with water over a high heat and bring to the boil. Add the eggs and cook for 5 minutes (for runny yolks). Cool under cold running water, then gently tap the eggs all over and carefully remove the shells. Set aside.

2. Place the onion rings and the oil in a large frying pan over a medium heat and fry until golden brown. Remove with a slotted spoon and set aside.

3. Add the diced onion to the pan and fry gently over a low heat for about 2 minutes.

4. Stir in the curry powder, bay leaves, if using, and fish, then pour in the milk to cover. Bring to a simmer. Add the raisins, grated cauliflower, courgette and chia seeds, cover and simmer for 5 minutes, until the fish is cooked through.

5. Remove and discard the bay leaves, and stir in the parsley and lemon juice. Gently break up the cooked fish and season generously with freshly ground black pepper. Serve with the eggs halved and placed on top, and the whole dish sprinkled with the onion rings.

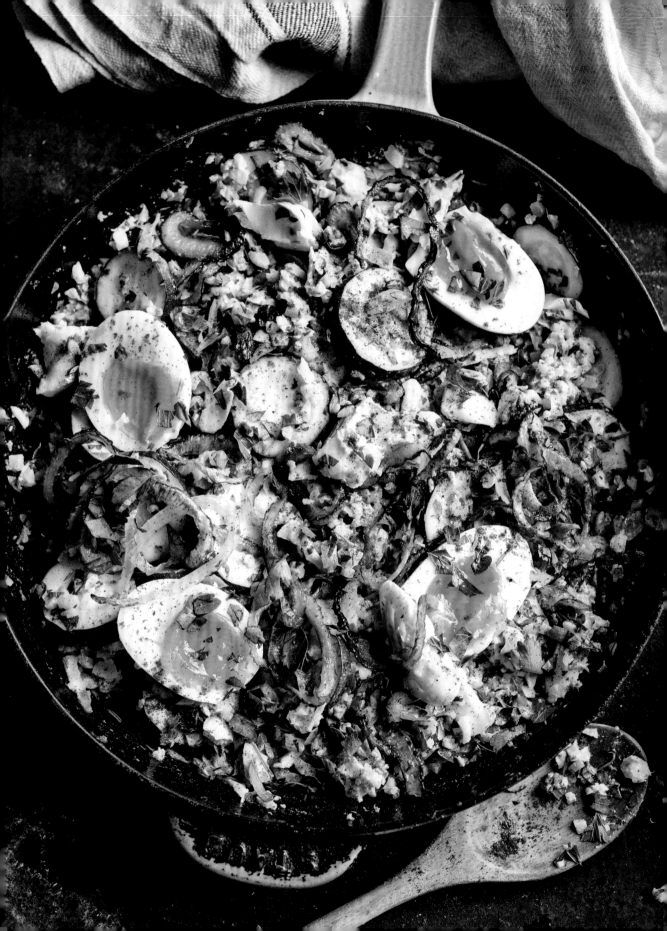

PER SERVING | **316cals** | PROTEIN **17.1g** | CARBS **4.8g**

Breakfast Burrito

SERVES	PREP	COOK
1	**5** mins	**15** mins

1 chipolata sausage,
   halved lengthways
2 rashers smoked
   streaky bacon
1 large mushroom,
   thinly sliced
2 cherry tomatoes, halved
1 tsp olive oil
1 medium free-range egg
2 large leaves iceberg lettuce
½ tsp full-fat mayonnaise
½ tsp sriracha (optional)

NON-FAST DAY
Serve a double portion.

A Mexican-inspired burrito cleverly served in crunchy lettuce.

1. Preheat the oven to 200°C/Fan 180°C/Gas 6 and line a baking tray with baking parchment.

2. Place the sausage, bacon, mushroom and tomatoes on the prepared tray. Drizzle the mushrooms and tomatoes with the oil, season with salt and freshly ground black pepper and roast in the oven for 12 minutes.

3. Remove the tray from the oven and make some space. Crack in the egg and return to the oven for a further 3 minutes.

4. To assemble, layer the iceberg leaves on top of one another, then spread with the mayo and sriracha (if using). Stack the cooked ingredients on top, roll tightly and serve.

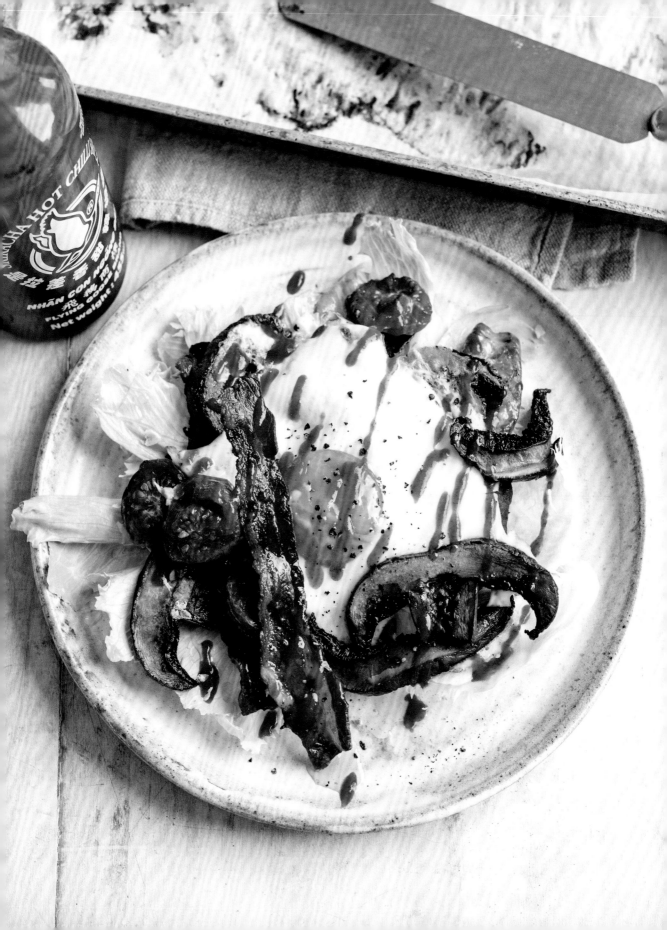

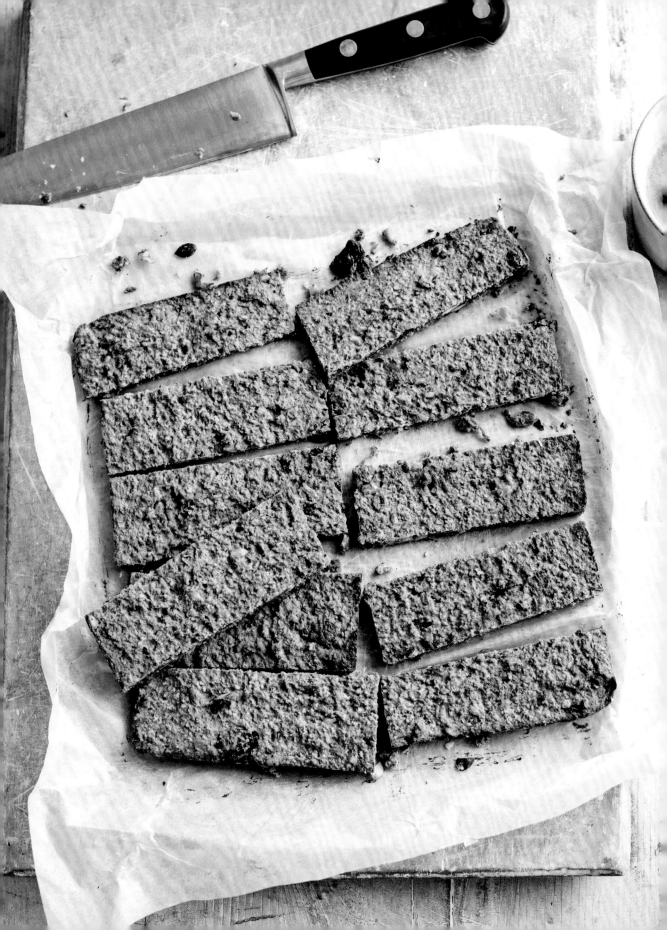

Cinnamon and Pecan Breakfast Bars

MAKES
12

PREP
15
mins

COOK
20
mins

3 medjool dates, destoned
   and cut into small pieces
   (approx. 55g)
1 tbsp coconut oil
1 tbsp vanilla extract
100g rolled oats
35g mix of pumpkin and
   sunflower seeds
10g dried cranberries
50g pecan nuts,
   roughly chopped
2 tsp ground cinnamon
1 level tbsp chia seeds
1 medium free-range egg

COOK'S TIP
These keep for up to 5 days
in an airtight container.

These versatile, nutty, high-fibre bars are ideal as a
breakfast on the go or for when you are out and about.
You could also crumble them into a bowl with 1–2
tablespoons full-fat yoghurt, but remember to add
the extra calories.

1. Preheat the oven to 200°C/Fan 180°C/Gas 6 and line
a 20cm square baking tin with baking parchment.

2. Place the dates in a deep bowl with the coconut oil and
100ml boiling water. Leave the dates to soften for 5 minutes.

3. Add the vanilla extract and blitz with a stick blender
until smooth.

4. In a separate bowl mix the oats, seeds, cranberries, pecan
nuts, cinnamon and a pinch of salt. Add the chia seeds to
the date mixture, then stir this into the dry mixture. Add
the egg and mix so that everything is thoroughly combined.

5. Transfer to the prepared tin and press the mixture down
firmly with a spatula. Bake in the oven for 10 minutes.
Remove from the oven, cut into 12 squares and leave
to cool in the tin.

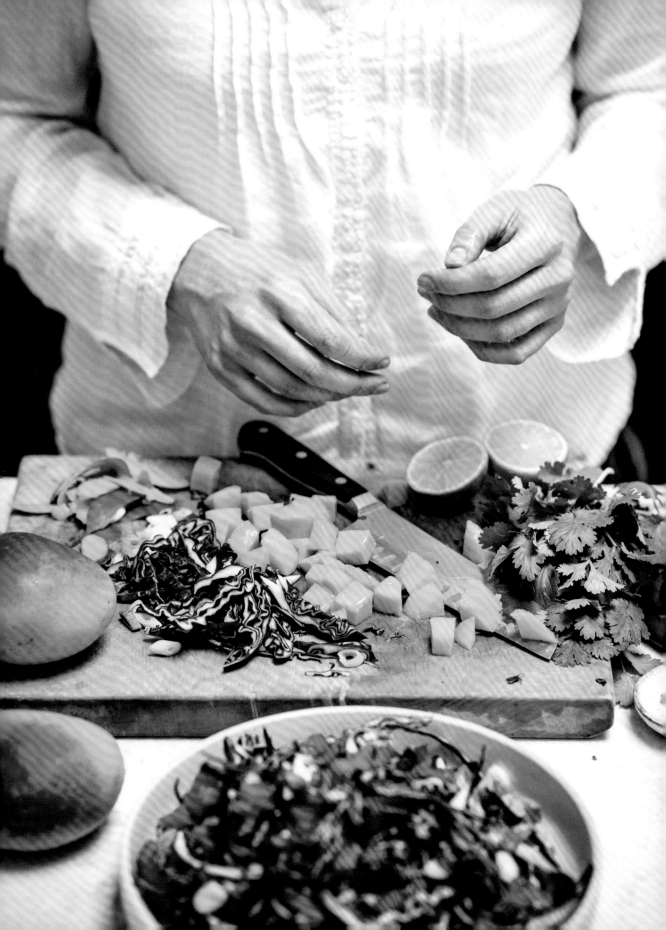

Light Bites & Lunch

Everyone eats their meals on a fast day differently. If you prefer to eat main meals at breakfast and dinner, you will find these light bites are just the thing to get you through the middle of the day. We have also included some great recipes for portable food to take to work or eat on the go.

PER SERVING | **253cals** | PROTEIN **38.3g** | CARBS **0.5g**

Chicken and Egg Noodle Soup

SERVES	PREP	COOK
2	**5** mins	**15** mins

1 chicken stock cube
1 garlic clove, peeled
   and finely chopped
2 medium free-range eggs
1 tsp olive oil
30g fresh spinach or
   cooked greens
200g cooked chicken, diced
10g fresh coriander or
   parsley, roughly chopped

COOK'S TIP
A few drops of sriracha
would be lovely in this broth
if you like a bit of heat.

NON-FAST DAY
Add wholemeal noodles
and/or edamame beans.

Few things are as comforting and satisfying as a bowl of chicken soup. These 'egg noodles' are made simply by cooking whisked eggs, as you would a pancake, then slicing them into thin noodles.

1. Place the stock cube, garlic and 500ml water in a saucepan and bring to the boil. Reduce the heat to low.

2. Meanwhile, whisk the eggs and add a pinch of salt and some freshly ground black pepper.

3. Heat the olive oil in a non-stick frying pan over a medium heat and pour in the eggs. Swirl them around to cover the bottom of the pan as you would with a pancake, then cook for 1–2 minutes, or until they are set. Transfer the egg 'pancake' to a clean surface, roll up and slice into thin noodles.

4. Add the spinach and chicken to the stock in the saucepan and simmer for 2–3 minutes.

5. Divide the egg 'noodles' between two bowls and pour over the chicken broth. Garnish with fresh coriander or parsley to serve.

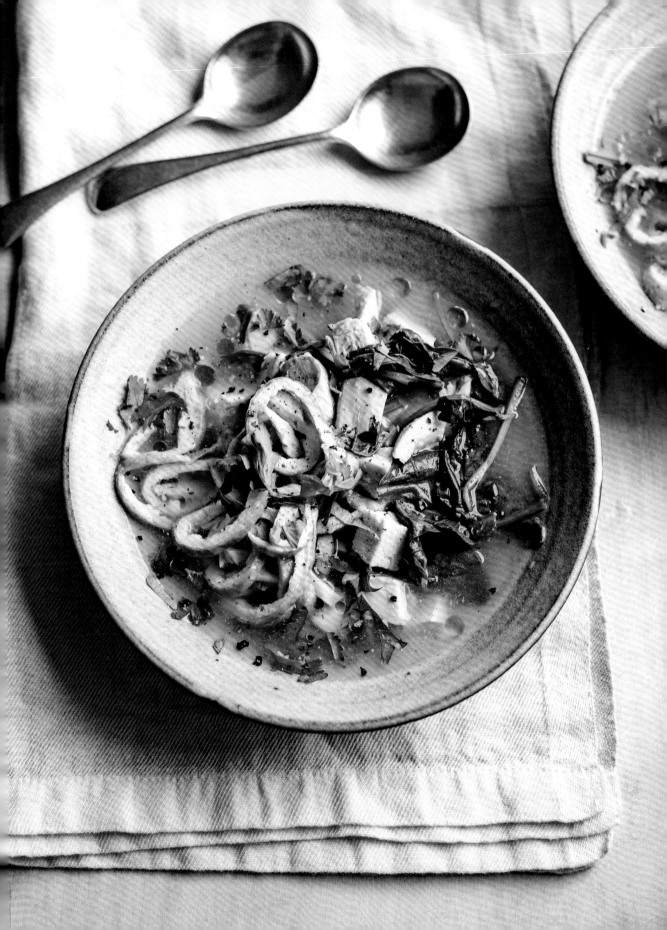

Low-carb Minestrone

SERVES	PREP	COOK
2	**10** mins	**10** mins

1 small onion, peeled
    and finely chopped
1 stick celery, finely chopped
1½ tbsp olive oil
2 garlic cloves, peeled
    and finely chopped
1 tbsp tomato purée
500ml chicken stock
    (made with 1 stock cube)
1 small red pepper
40g edamame beans
200g cooked chicken,
    finely chopped
30g Parmesan, finely grated

NON-FAST DAY
Serve with a slice of seeded
sourdough or wholemeal
bread for dipping.

Remarkably high in protein and nutrients for a simple soup, this will power you through the day. Protein really is key, keeping you feeling full for longer and supporting lots of vital functions. The tragedy is that most of us are not getting enough of it in our daily diet.

1. Place the onion, celery and olive oil in a saucepan over a low heat and sauté for 4 minutes, stirring occasionally. Add the garlic and cook for 1 minute more.

2. Stir in the tomato purée, followed by the stock and bring to the boil.

3. Reduce to a simmer and add the red pepper, edamame beans and cooked chicken. Cook for 3–4 minutes.

4. Remove from the heat and add the Parmesan. It will melt instantly and give the soup a lovely creamy texture. Season with freshly ground black pepper and serve.

Cajun Cauliflower Soup with Silken Tofu

SERVES	PREP	COOK
4	**5–7** mins	**25** mins

1 leek, trimmed and
    roughly sliced
2 garlic cloves, peeled
    and roughly chopped
½ red chilli, chopped
    (optional)
2 tbsp olive oil
1 cauliflower, broken into
    florets (approx. 400g
    prepared weight)
1 tbsp Cajun seasoning
1.2 litres vegetable stock
    (made using 2 stock cubes)
200g silken tofu

COOK'S TIPS
Any leftover tofu from
the packet can be used
in the French Dressing
with Tofu (see page 237).
If you are not adding chilli,
increase the amount
of Cajun seasoning to
1½ tablespoons.

NON-FAST DAY
Serve with a slice of
sourdough or wholemeal
bread for dipping.

A mildly spiced, creamy, yet very low-calorie soup.
You could add another layer of texture and a boost of
protein, by including a protein top-up (see page 240)
such as grated Cheddar, fried chorizo or toasted
sunflower seeds. Adding this kind of keto-friendly
top-up is OK, and you don't need to worry about
the extra calories.

1. Place the leek, garlic, chilli, if using, and olive oil in a
saucepan over a medium heat and sauté for 5–6 minutes,
stirring from time to time.

2. Add the cauliflower florets, Cajun seasoning and
stock and bring to the boil. Reduce the heat and simmer
for 20 minutes.

3. Remove from the heat, add the tofu and blitz with a
stick blender until completely smooth. Season with salt
and freshly ground black pepper to serve.

PER SERVING | **293cals** | PROTEIN **5.1g** | CARBS **6.9g**

Creamy Broccoli, Ginger and Coriander Soup

SERVES **4** | PREP **5–7** mins | COOK **15–20** mins

1 small onion, peeled and
   roughly chopped
40g fresh root ginger, roughly
   chopped (no need to peel)
1½ tbsp olive oil
1 head of broccoli,
   roughly chopped
1 × 400ml tin coconut milk
1 vegetable stock cube
15g fresh coriander
40g flaked almonds,
   toasted, to garnish

COOK'S TIP
Add a protein top-up,
if you like (see page 240).
Fried diced bacon or feta
cheese would go well.

A light soup with the warming qualities of coconut, ginger and coriander running through it. The recipe makes enough for four, but it keeps well in the fridge or freezer.

1. Place the onion, ginger and olive oil in a large saucepan over a medium heat and sauté for 3–4 minutes, until softened.

2. Add the broccoli, coconut milk, stock cube and 800ml water (simply refill the empty coconut milk tin twice). Bring to the boil, reduce the heat and simmer for 10 minutes.

3. Remove from the heat, add the coriander and blitz with a stick blender until completely smooth. Season with salt and freshly ground black pepper and serve, topped with flaked almonds.

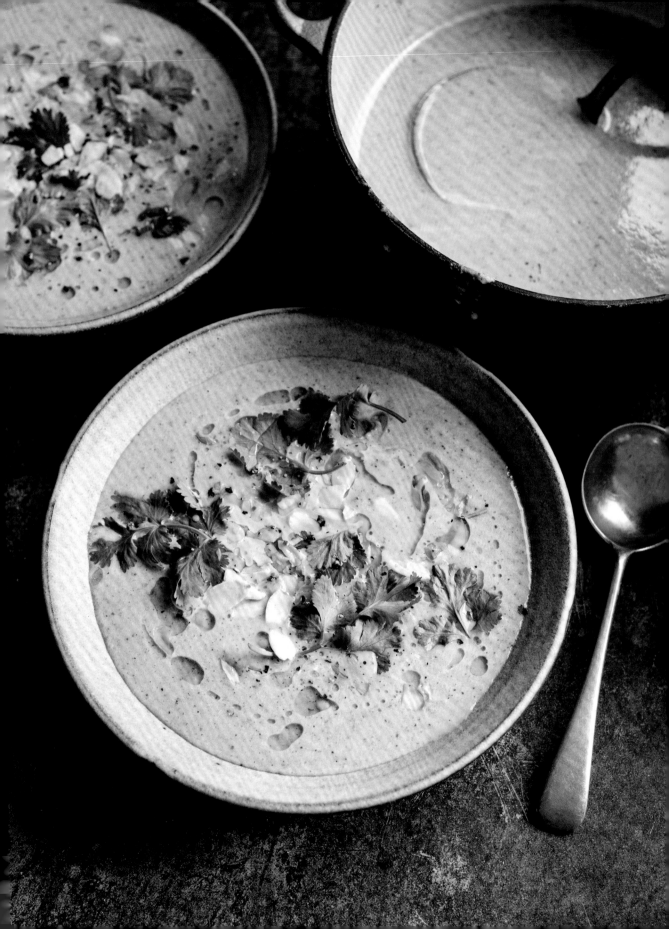

PER SERVING | **332cals** | PROTEIN **11.3g** | CARBS **27.5g**

Black Bean and Mango Slaw

SERVES | PREP
2 | **30**
  | mins

½ × 400g tin black beans,
    drained and rinsed
    (approx. 120g drained weight)
1 medium red pepper, deseeded
    and cut into 1cm pieces
¼ small red cabbage, core
    removed and finely sliced
2–3 spring onions, trimmed
    and finely chopped
30g pine nuts
½ mango, diced (approx. 150g
    prepared weight)
2 generous handfuls rocket
    or watercress
1 small red chilli, finely sliced
    (deseeded, if preferred,
    for less heat)
Small handful coriander,
    roughly chopped (optional)

For the dressing:
1 tbsp fresh lime juice
2 tbsp full-fat Greek yoghurt
1 tbsp full-fat mayo

COOK'S TIP
You can use two halves of
apricot or one peach from
a tin (approx. 100g) instead
of mango, if you wish.

Although the beans and mango make this salad slightly
higher in carbs than other slaws, these ingredients
really make the salad sing! The beans also offer vital
extra fibre to help feed your gut microbiome – which in
turn supports your immunity, reduces inflammation,
boosts mood and may even help with weight loss.

1. Mix the black beans, red pepper, red cabbage and spring
onions together in a large bowl.

2. Toast the pine nuts in a dry frying pan over a medium
heat for about 2 minutes, until they start to turn golden.
Be careful they don't burn.

3. To make the dressing, place half the mango in a jug
with the lime juice, yoghurt and mayo and blitz with a stick
blender. Season with salt and freshly ground black pepper.

4. Stir the dressing into the beans and veg, then gently
toss in the leaves. Divide between two plates and top with
the remaining mango. Garnish with the pine nuts, chilli
and coriander, if using, to serve.

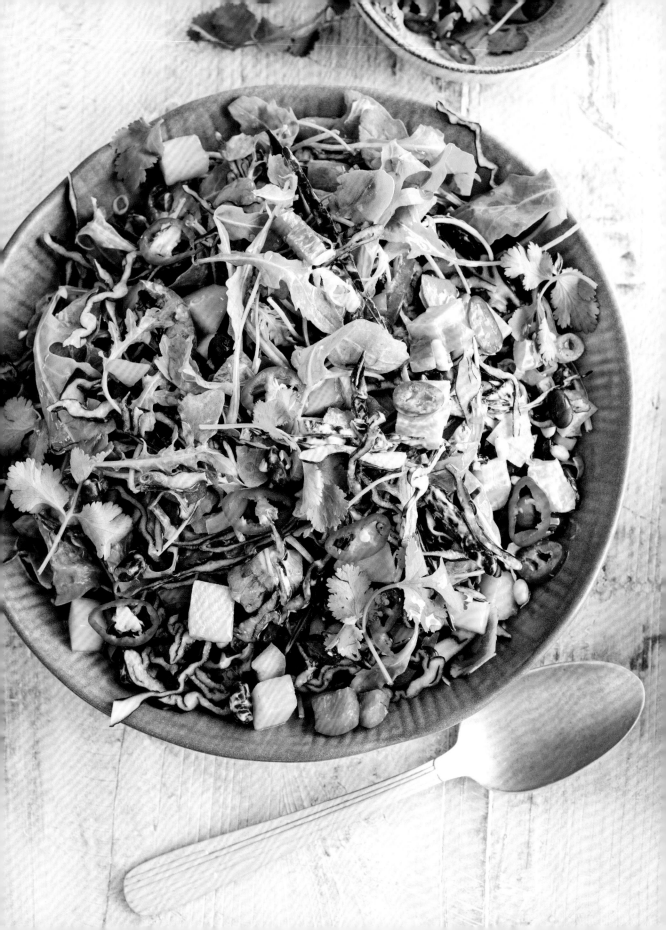

PER SERVING | **285cals** | PROTEIN **13.4g** | CARBS **1.3g**

Warm Crispy Kale Salad with Mushrooms, Bacon and Goat's Cheese

SERVES	PREP	COOK
2	**8** mins	**12** mins

125g curly kale, hard stems
   stripped out and leaves
   roughly chopped
2 tbsp olive oil
½–1 tsp chilli flakes
2 large Portobello mushrooms,
   finely sliced
4 rashers smoked streaky
   bacon, snipped into pieces
50g soft goat's cheese

COOK'S TIP

Keep a close eye on the kale
to make sure it doesn't burn.

NON-FAST DAY

Have an extra half portion,
and serve on toasted
wholemeal bread or
seeded sourdough.

Kale cooked in the oven becomes irresistibly crispy.
Eat this salad in a wide bowl.

1. Preheat the oven to 200°C/Fan 180°C/Gas 6.

2. Tip the kale into a roasting dish, drizzle with 1 tablespoon
of the olive oil, sprinkle over the chilli flakes and season
with salt and freshly ground black pepper. Using both
hands, massage the oil into the leaves so they are
thoroughly coated. Roast in the oven for 5 minutes.

3. Meanwhile, place the mushrooms, bacon and remaining
oil in a pan over a medium heat and sauté for about 5 minutes,
until starting to brown and crisp. Remove from the heat.

4. To assemble, divide the kale, bacon and mushrooms
between two bowls. Dot the goat's cheese all over and serve.

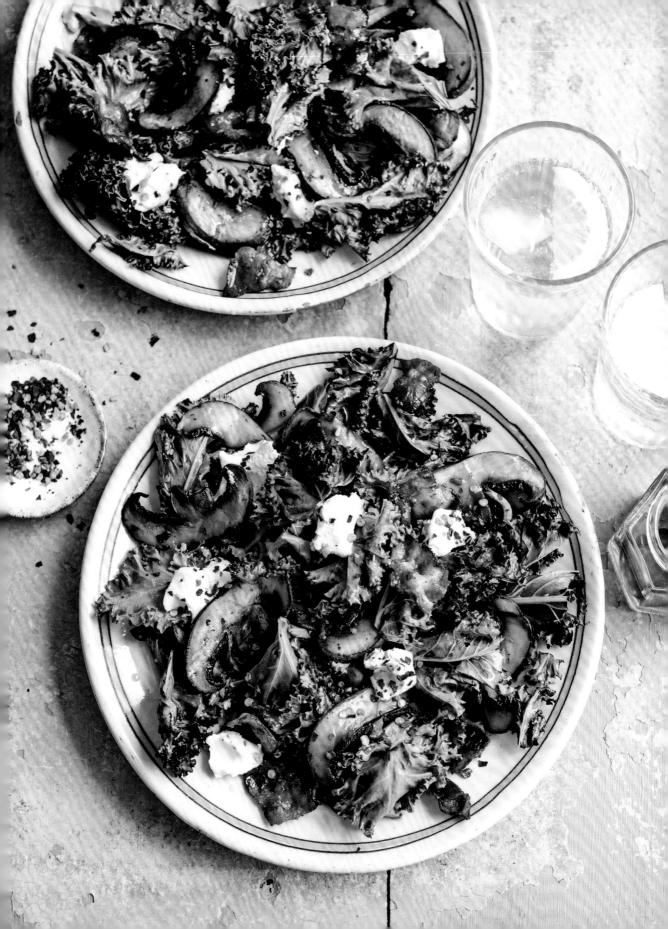

PER SERVING | **502cals** | PROTEIN **35.1g** | CARBS **17.5g**

Mixed Bean and Miso Salad with Chicken

SERVES | PREP
2 | **10** mins

1 red or orange pepper,
    deseeded and finely chopped
1 spring onion, trimmed
    and finely chopped
100g frozen edamame
    beans, defrosted
150g cooked chicken,
    finely chopped
½ × 400g tin mixed beans
50g fresh spinach,
    roughly chopped
1 portion Miso Dressing
    (see page 236)

NON-FAST DAY
Stir in 2–3 tablespoons
cooked quinoa or brown
rice, or serve with a slice of
toasted seeded sourdough
or wholemeal bread.

A vibrant, tangy salad, which offers a generous portion and is high in protein and gut-friendly fibre to keep you feeling full. It also makes a great lunchbox salad.

1. Combine all the ingredients in a bowl and mix well.

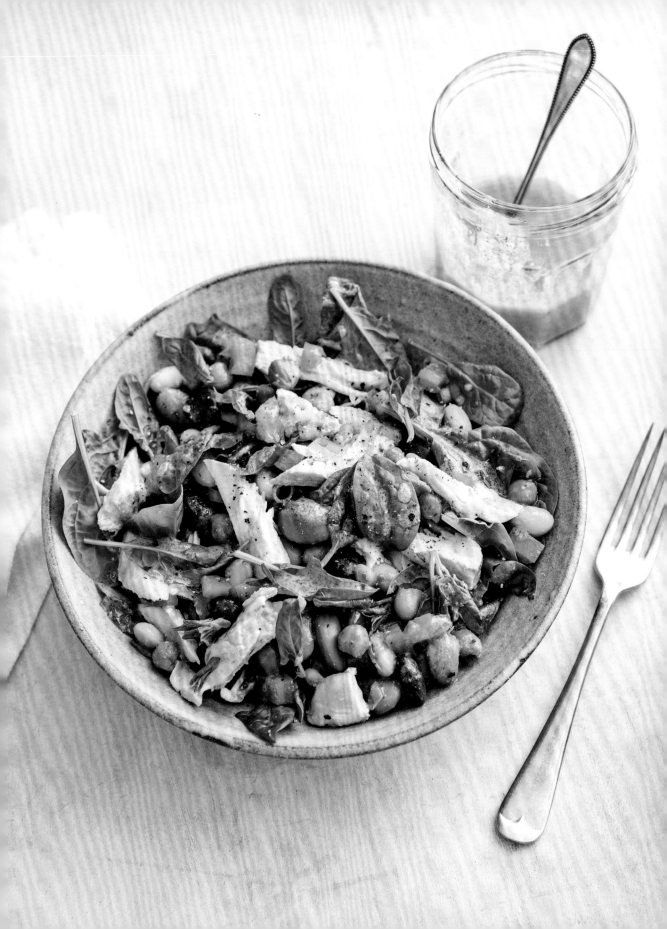

Warm Smoked Mackerel Salad with Mustard Dressing

SERVES **2** | **PREP** **10** mins | **COOK** **10** mins

2 cooked smoked mackerel
   fillets (approx. 140g total
   weight), skin removed
   and flaked
150g broccoli, broken
   into florets
40g cooked Puy lentils
50g salad leaves
2 tsp capers

For the dressing:
1 heaped tsp wholegrain
   mustard
1 tbsp cider vinegar
2 tbsp olive oil

COOK'S TIP
Cooked Puy lentils and
cooked mackerel fillets
are available in most
supermarkets. Mackerel
comes in different flavours,
including sweet chilli
and peppered.

NON-FAST DAY
Serve a larger portion.

Mackerel is a fabulous and affordable high-protein superfood, offering you a healthy dose of anti-inflammatory omega-3. The robust dressing works really well here.

1. Remove the mackerel from the fridge a few minutes ahead, as they are best served at room temperature.

2. Place the dressing ingredients in a small jar with a lid and shake briefly until the dressing thickens. Set aside.

3. Steam or boil the broccoli in a little salted water until just tender. Heat the lentils briefly so they are warmed (microwave is fine).

4. Divide the salad leaves between two plates. Top with the lentils, broccoli, flaked mackerel fillets and capers. Season with salt and freshly ground pepper and drizzle the dressing all over to serve.

Creamy Egg Salad

SERVES **2** | PREP **5** mins | COOK **8** mins

4 medium free-range eggs
1 tbsp mayonnaise
1 tbsp full-fat Greek yoghurt
5 cherry tomatoes, quartered
2 spring onions, trimmed
    and finely chopped
40g rocket, roughly chopped

NON-FAST DAY
Serve with seeded sourdough
or wholemeal bread.

If you have calories to spare, serve with Instant
Mug Bread (see page 206).

1. Bring a medium saucepan of water to the boil, add the
eggs and cook for 8 minutes. Drain and run the eggs under
cold water to stop them from cooking. Peel and cut each
egg into quarters.

2. Meanwhile, combine the mayonnaise and Greek yoghurt
in a medium bowl and season with salt and freshly ground
black pepper.

3. Add the eggs to the bowl along with the tomatoes,
spring onions and rocket and mix well.

Stuffed Mini Peppers

SERVES **2** | PREP **10** mins | COOK **12** mins

6 mini peppers or 2 small
    peppers, halved, deseeded
    but stem retained
120g cooked chicken,
    finely chopped
50g Cheddar, grated
2 tsp fajita seasoning
1 portion Sriracha Yoghurt
    Dressing (see page 236)

NON-FAST DAY
Serve a double portion.

These Mexican-flavoured, stuffed mini peppers are
ideal for a quick light lunch. They would also work well
shared on a platter, or scattered on to a generous salad.

1. Preheat the oven to 200°C/Fan 180°C/Gas 6 and line
a baking tray with baking parchment.

2. Place the peppers cut-side-up on the tray.

3. Mix the chicken, Cheddar and fajita seasoning together
in a small bowl. Season with salt and freshly ground black
pepper. Stuff the peppers with the chicken mixture,
pressing down well, and bake in the oven for 12 minutes.

4. Drizzle Sriracha Yoghurt Dressing over the top to serve.

Sardines with Roasted Red Peppers

SERVES
1

PREP
5
mins

100g roasted red peppers
   from a jar, finely chopped
100g cucumber, finely chopped
30g pitted black olives,
   roughly chopped
5g flat-leaf parsley,
   roughly chopped
1½ tsp balsamic vinegar
1 × 95g tin sardines in
   olive oil, drained

NON-FAST DAY
Serve the peppers and
sardines on toasted
brown sourdough or
wholemeal bread.

This recipe is a simple assembly job, no cooking required. It is sunshine on a plate, full of deliciously satisfying Mediterranean flavours and bursting with healthy omega-3. It serves one but can easily be scaled up.

1. Mix the roasted red peppers, cucumber, black olives, parsley and 1 teaspoon of the balsamic vinegar together in a bowl. Season well with salt and freshly ground black pepper.

2. Remove the sardines from the tin and serve them on top of the salad. Drizzle the remaining balsamic all over, check the seasoning and serve.

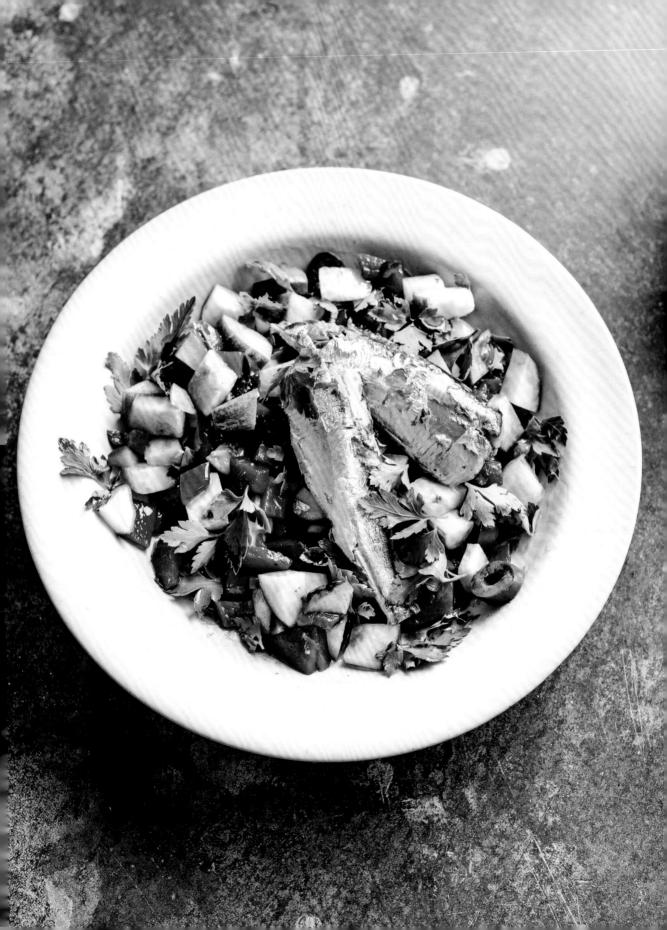

Broccoli Fritters with Eggs and Bacon

SERVES **2** | PREP **10** mins | COOK **10–15** mins

¼ **head of broccoli, finely chopped including the stalk**
2 rashers smoked back bacon
1½ tbsp olive oil
4 level tbsp ground almonds
40g Cheddar, grated
4 medium free-range eggs

COOK'S TIP
For bite-sized snacks, make smaller fritters. When cooked and cooled, these can be kept in an airtight container in the fridge for up to 3 days. If you don't have a microwave, steam the broccoli florets for 3–4 minutes, then chop finely.

NON-FAST DAY
Increase the portion size, or add 2–3 tablespoons wholegrain rice and/or sliced avocado.

Broccoli fritters are wonderfully filling when served with eggs and bacon, but also make great fridge-ready snacks on their own. If you have any herbs to hand, such as dill or parsley, they would add extra flavour.

1. Place the broccoli in a microwave-safe glass bowl with 1 tablespoon of water, cover and microwave for 1½ minutes. Leave to cool slightly but don't drain the water.

2. Meanwhile, place the bacon and ½ tablespoon of the olive oil in a non-stick frying pan and fry for 3–4 minutes, depending on how crispy you like it. Set aside and keep warm.

3. Add the ground almonds, Cheddar and 2 of the eggs to the broccoli and stir. Season well with salt and freshly ground black pepper.

4. Pour the remaining oil into the frying pan and place over a medium heat. When the oil is hot, scrape the broccoli mixture into the pan to make two fritters. Flatten them slightly and cook for 1½–2 minutes on each side.

5. Remove the fritters from the pan and keep warm. Add a splash more oil to the pan, if necessary, and crack in the remaining eggs. Cook to your liking, then stack the fried eggs on the broccoli fritters and top with the bacon to serve.

Green Protein Wraps

SERVES	PREP	COOK
2	**5** mins	**5** mins

2 medium free-range eggs
1 tbsp wholegrain flour
10g Parmesan, finely grated
50g frozen spinach,
    defrosted and excess
    liquid squeezed out
1 tsp olive oil

COOK'S TIP
The batter will keep for
a day in the fridge so you
can use half and keep
the remaining batter
for the next day.

These high-protein wraps are a brilliant vehicle for all
sorts of delicious fillings and will seamlessly replace
carb-heavy sandwiches.

1. Place the eggs, flour, Parmesan and spinach in a bowl
and blitz using a stick blender until smooth. Season with
a little salt and freshly ground black pepper.

2. Swirl ½ teaspoon of the oil around a non-stick frying
pan and place over a medium heat. Pour in half the batter
and tilt the pan to spread out. Fry for 45–60 seconds, then
carefully flip over. Fry for a further 30 seconds, then transfer
to a plate.

3. Repeat with the remaining batter.

4. Serve with a filling of your choice.

Curried Chicken Protein Wrap

SERVES	PREP
2	**5–7** mins

200g cooked chicken, diced
1 portion Curried Yoghurt
    Dressing (see page 237)
2 Green Protein Wraps
    (see above)
50g iceberg lettuce
10g Cheddar, grated

You can take this creamy chicken wrap anywhere;
or just enjoy it at home, rolled and sliced into
bite-sized pieces. If you are making this for one,
keep the remaining curried chicken in the fridge
to use the following day.

1. Mix the chicken with the Curried Yoghurt Dressing.

2. Divide between the wraps and top with the iceberg
lettuce and cheese to serve.

PER SERVING | **253cals** | PROTEIN **18.9g** | CARBS **6.6g**

Sriracha Prawn Cocktail Protein Wrap

SERVES | PREP
2 | **5–7**
mins

150g cooked and peeled prawns
1 portion Sriracha Yoghurt
   Dressing (see page 236)
½ small avocado, peeled,
   stoned and roughly
   chopped (approx. 50g
   prepared weight)
Squeeze of lime
50g cucumber, cut into
   1cm dice
2 Green Protein Wraps
   (see page 65)

COOK'S TIP
Frozen cooked prawns
can be used, but defrost
them first and drain off
any excess water.

NON-FAST DAY
Serve a double portion.

Prawn cocktail in a wrap – very retro, but still indulgent.If you are making this for one, you can keep the remaining prawns in the fridge until the following day.

1. Mix the prawns with the Sriracha Yoghurt Dressing and season with salt and freshly ground black pepper.

2. Toss the avocado with a squeeze of lime juice.

3. Divide the ingredients between the wraps and serve.

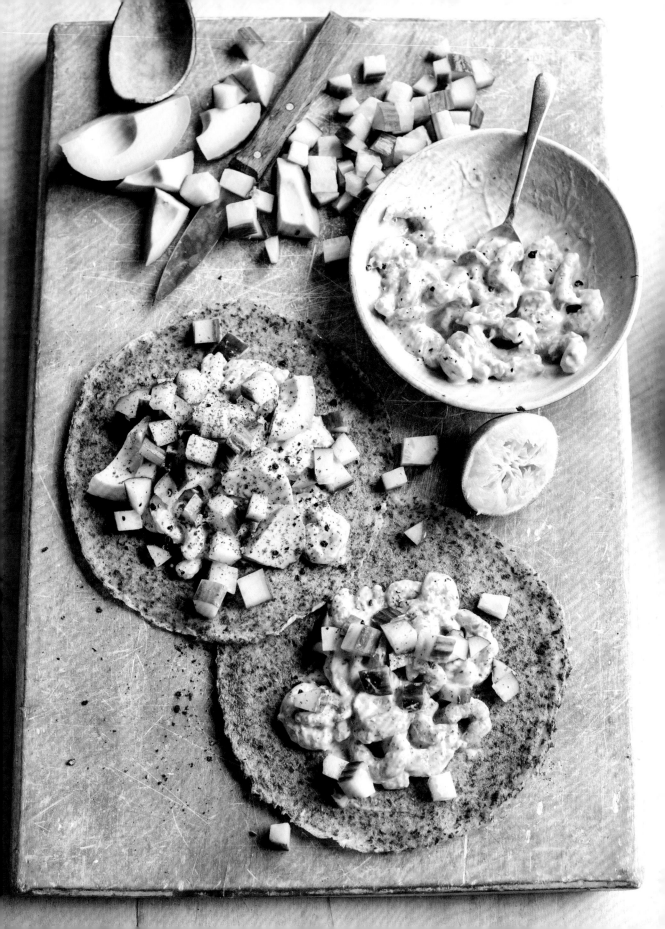

PER SERVING | **427cals** | PROTEIN **24.4g** | CARBS **16.6g**

Pink Cauli Risotto with Halloumi and Spinach

SERVES	PREP	COOK
2	**10** mins	**8–10** mins

1 small onion, peeled
    and finely chopped
100g chestnut
    mushrooms, sliced
1 tbsp olive oil
100g halloumi, diced
250g cauli-rice (see TIP)
200ml vegetable stock
    (made using ½ veg
    stock cube)
1 tbsp chia seeds
100g frozen spinach,
    defrosted
25g Parmesan, grated
1 tbsp crème fraîche
50g cooked beetroot,
    peeled and diced
Juice of ½ lemon

COOK'S TIP
Make cauli-rice by grating
or quickly blitzing half a
cauliflower, or buy it ready-
made from the supermarket
freezer cabinet.

NON-FAST DAY
Add a protein top-up of
your choice, such as toasted
seeds, edamame or diced
ham or chorizo.

This super-quick yet lusciously creamy risotto swaps
starchy risotto rice for cauli-rice. The trick here is that
we use chia seeds to help thicken the sauce and create
a smooth, silky texture. The beetroot adds a gorgeous
pink colour – and can help reduce blood pressure and
fight inflammation.

1. Place the onion, mushrooms and oil in a saucepan and
sauté for 2 minutes. Add the halloumi and fry for 2 minutes
more, or until the halloumi starts to take on some colour.

2. Stir in the cauliflower rice, stock and chia seeds and cook,
stirring often, for 3–4 minutes, until some of the stock has
reduced and thickened slightly.

3. Stir in the spinach, Parmesan and crème fraîche, and
season to taste with salt and freshly ground black pepper.

4. Fold in the beetroot, squeeze over the lemon juice
and serve immediately.

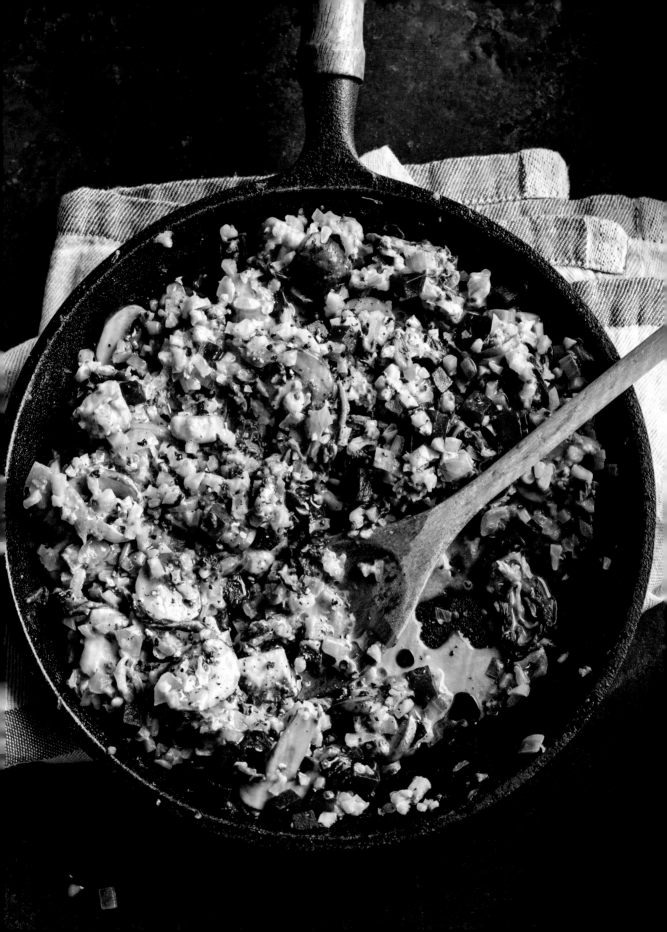

PER SERVING | **382cals** | PROTEIN **44.1g** | CARBS **13g**

Cauli-rice Risotto with Chicken, Asparagus and Tarragon

SERVES | PREP | COOK
2 | **15** mins | **10** mins

1 small onion, peeled
  and finely chopped
4 garlic cloves, peeled
  and finely chopped
1 tbsp olive oil
250g cauli-rice (see page 68)
70g asparagus, woody
  ends removed, spears
  finely chopped
1 heaped tsp dried tarragon
1 tbsp chia seeds
250ml chicken stock
  (made using ½ stock cube)
250g cooked chicken,
  roughly chopped
1 tbsp crème fraîche

COOK'S TIP
If you don't have any cooked
chicken, finely slice 2
boneless, skinless chicken
thighs and fry in 1 tablespoon
of olive oil for 7 minutes
prior to starting the recipe.

You could replace the
chicken with fried halloumi
for a meat-free version.

NON-FAST DAY
Have a larger portion
and/or add grated Parmesan.

This speedy cauliflower risotto is deliciously creamy
thanks to the chia seeds, which have magical thickening
properties. The garlic marries beautifully with the
classic combination of chicken, asparagus and tarragon.
Serve with a generous colourful salad.

1. Place the onion, garlic and olive oil in a large pan over a
medium heat and sauté for 4–5 minutes, until soft and just
beginning to take on some colour. If the onions start to
catch, add a splash of water.

2. Stir in the cauliflower rice and cook for 1 minute.
Add the asparagus, dried tarragon, chia seeds and chicken
stock. Mix everything well and cook over a high heat for
about 5 minutes, stirring all the time to encourage some
of the liquid to reduce and the sauce to thicken.

3. Reduce the heat and add the cooked chicken and crème
fraîche. Gently warm through, making sure not to let the
crème fraîche boil. Season to taste with salt and freshly
ground black pepper.

Courgetti with Prawns and Creamy Garlic Sauce

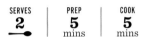

SERVES	PREP	COOK
2	**5** mins	**5** mins

2 tbsp olive oil

250g large peeled prawns, defrosted

Zest of 1 lemon

½ tsp chilli flakes, to taste (optional)

2 medium courgettes, spiralised or julienned

75g Garlic and Herb Boursin

NON-FAST DAY

Add 20–40g wholemeal, green or yellow pea pasta.

Courgetti is your keto saviour – enabling you to enjoy these fabulous pasta flavours with minimal carbs and calories.

1. Heat the oil in a frying pan over a high heat. When hot, add the prawns, lemon zest and chilli flakes, if using, and cook for 1–2 minutes, stirring occasionally.

2. Reduce the heat to medium and add the courgetti. Cook for about 1 minute, until warmed through, stirring regularly.

3. Stir in the Boursin and add 1 tablespoon of water to loosen, if needed (the sauce should be a creamy consistency). Season with salt and freshly ground black pepper to serve.

PER SERVING | **331cals** | PROTEIN **12.5g** | CARBS **6.6g**

Pesto Courgetti Spaghetti with Red Pepper and Feta

SERVES	PREP	COOK
2	**10** mins	**10** mins

2 tbsp olive oil
2 roasted red peppers
  from a jar, sliced
2 medium courgettes,
  spiralised or julienned
2 tbsp pesto, red or green
100g feta cheese, diced
15g pine nuts
Small handful basil
  leaves (optional)

COOK'S TIP
For extra flavour and protein, add a couple of tablespoons diced cooked bacon or chorizo and a pinch of chilli flakes.

NON-FAST DAY
Cook 40g pasta according to the packet instructions. Just before the pasta is ready, add the spiralised courgette to the pan and cook until the water returns to the boil (usually 30–60 seconds). Drain immediately and reserve 2–3 tablespoons of the cooking liquid to loosen the sauce. Add to the pan with the peppers and continue to cook as above.

A quick, tasty lunch you can throw together at the last minute. Apart from the courgette, most of the ingredients can be found in your cupboard, where they retain their freshness and nutrients. This dish works for the whole family – just add some spaghetti (ideally wholemeal) and offer larger portions.

1. Place the oil in a large frying pan over a medium heat. Add the peppers and heat through for 1–2 minutes, stirring occasionally.

2. Add the courgetti and cook, stirring, for about 1 minute.

3. Stir in the pesto and feta. Heat through and add a tablespoon of water, if needed, to loosen.

4. Scatter with the pine nuts and the basil leaves, if using, and season with plenty of freshly ground black pepper to serve.

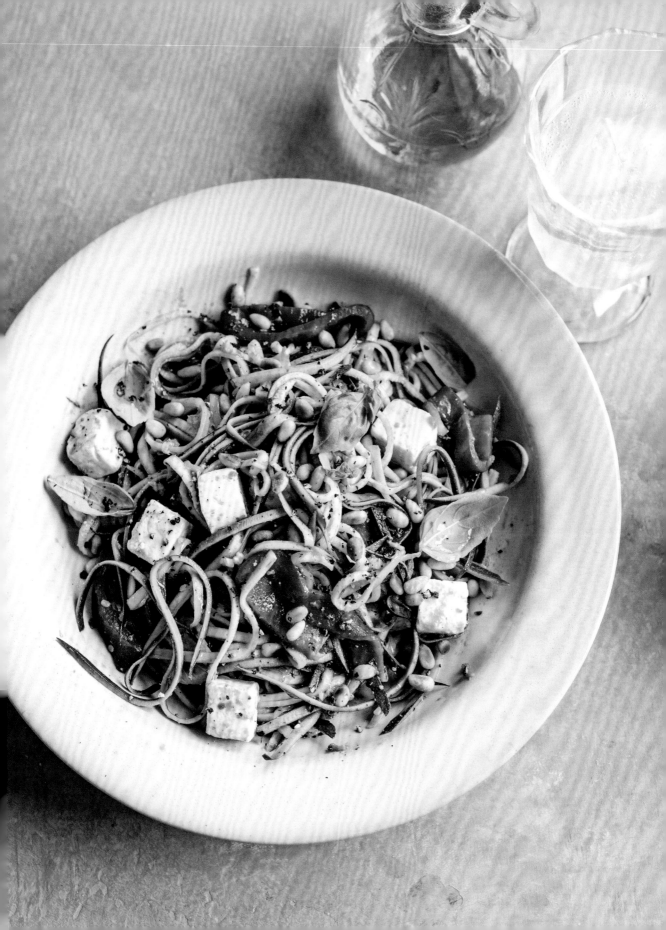

One Pan Creamy Cabbage Pappardelle with Walnuts and Gorgonzola

SERVES	PREP	COOK
2	**10** mins	**10** mins

30g walnuts, roughly chopped
20g pumpkin seeds
1 tbsp olive oil
½ small pointed cabbage,
   core removed, sliced into
   0.5cm-wide strips
70g crème fraîche
50g Gorgonzola, roughly diced
1 tbsp cider vinegar
½ small conference pear,
   core removed and diced
   (no need to peel)
Pinch of chilli flakes (optional)

NON-FAST DAY
Add diced cooked chicken,
diced bacon, peas and/or
edamame beans.

This recipe was inspired by a restaurant meal of pasta, walnuts and Gorgonzola – a classic Italian combination, which I felt needed tweaking! Out went the heavy pasta – in came cabbage pappardelle and a lighter, zingier sauce, thanks to a little cider vinegar and some sweet, juicy pear. So easy and all cooked in one pan. For extra protein, you might want to add a slice of delicious, salty prosciutto (see protein top-ups on page 240).

1. Toast the walnuts in a large dry frying pan over a medium heat for 2–3 minutes, stirring occasionally, until golden brown in places. Set aside. Do the same with the pumpkin seeds, which will only need 1–2 minutes. Set aside with the walnuts.

2. Place the oil in the pan over a medium heat, add the cabbage and cook, stirring occasionally, for 3–4 minutes, until softened but with a little bite.

3. Meanwhile, place the crème fraîche, Gorgonzola and cider vinegar in a small bowl and mix well.

4. When the cabbage is almost cooked, stir in the Gorgonzola sauce and heat through. Add half the pear, mix well and divide between two bowls. Top with the remaining pear, the walnuts and pumpkin seeds and a pinch of chilli flakes, if using.

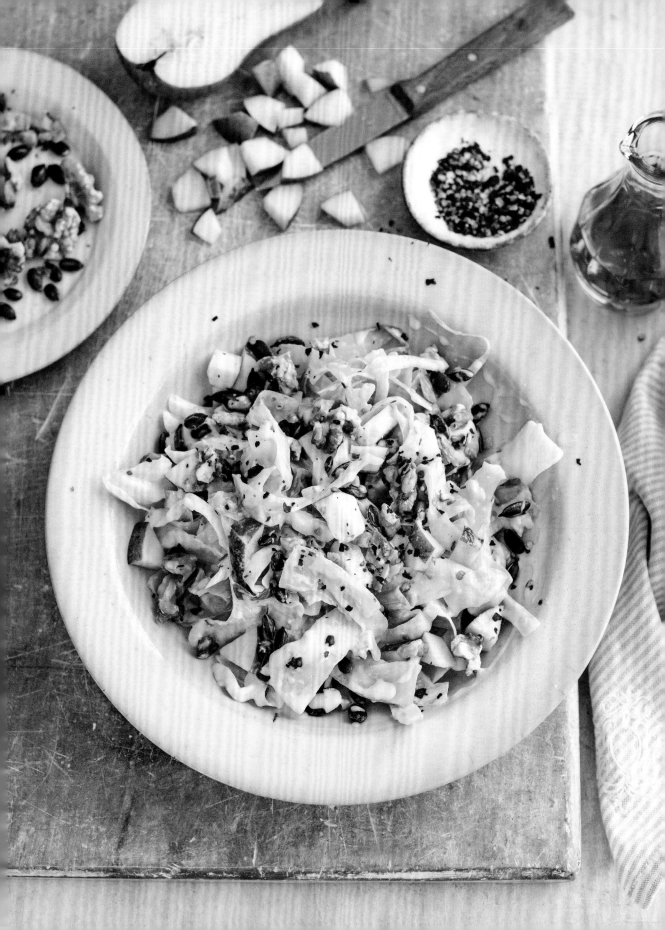

PER SERVING | **213cals** | PROTEIN **7.9g** | CARBS **3.7g**

Chicken Liver Pâté

SERVES **4** | PREP **2–3** mins | COOK **15–20** mins

100g butter
1 medium onion,
    peeled and diced
200g chicken livers
½ tsp dried thyme
2 garlic cloves, peeled
    and roughly chopped
1½ tbsp balsamic vinegar

NON-FAST DAY
Have an extra portion and
spread it on wholemeal toast
or pitta, topped with chilli
jam. Serve with a dressed
salad. You could also spread
it on Thin Seeded Chilli
Crackers (see page 201).

This is cheap and easy to make and highly nutritious.
Enjoy it as a dip with crunchy veg, or have it in a wrap
with salad and pickled veg.

1. Place a frying pan over a medium heat and melt the
butter. Add the onion and allow to sweat for 3–4 minutes,
then stir in the chicken livers and thyme. Cook, stirring
occasionally, for 7–8 minutes. Add the garlic and cook
for 2 minutes more.

2. Remove from the heat and add the balsamic vinegar
and plenty of freshly ground black pepper. Set aside
to cool for about 5 minutes.

3. Transfer to a deep bowl and blitz until smooth with
a stick blender. Alternatively, use a food processor.

4. Store in a lidded container and refrigerate until
required. It takes up to an hour to set in the fridge
and will keep for 4–5 days.

Leftover Chicken with Puy Lentils and Tomatoes

SERVES | PREP | COOK
2 | **5** mins | **5** mins

2 tbsp olive oil
1 small onion, peeled
   and diced
150g cooked chicken,
   roughly chopped
125g cherry tomatoes
1 tsp of Za'atar (or other
   dried herbs of choice)
125g cooked Puy lentils
1 tbsp cider vinegar
100g feta cheese, cut into
   1–2cm pieces

COOK'S TIP
You can swap the chicken
for a different protein,
such as fish (pre-cooked
and smoked would be ideal),
edamame beans or tofu.

NON-FAST DAY
Increase the portion size
and/or add some roast
butternut squash slices,
extra tomatoes and a
drizzle of olive oil.

It might sound as if we live on leftovers, and that's
partly true – we try to throw very little food away,
and often cook double portions for convenience.
This means keeping wholegrains, such as brown
rice or quinoa, as well as leftover cooked greens, in
the fridge or freezer, so they're ready when you need
them. Add some leftover chicken and you have an
almost-instant lunch.

1. Heat the oil in a frying pan and cook the onions
for 2–3 minutes over a medium heat, until softened.

2. Add the chicken, tomatoes and Za'atar and stir well.

3. Stir in the lentils and cider vinegar and cook for
3–4 minutes, stirring occasionally, then scatter the feta
over the top. Allow the feta to warm for 1–2 minutes,
then add a generous grind of black pepper to serve.

PER SERVING | **274cals** | PROTEIN **24.8g** | CARBS **3.4g**

Thai Pork Lettuce Cups

SERVES	PREP	COOK
2	**12** mins	**8** mins

1 tbsp olive oil
250g minced pork or chicken
1 stick lemongrass, 1cm
    removed from the base,
    tough outer layer removed,
    stem finely chopped
15g fresh root ginger,
    peeled and grated
2 garlic cloves, peeled
    and finely chopped
1 spring onion, finely sliced
4 baby gem lettuce leaves
Small handful coriander,
    leaves picked (optional)

For the dressing:
zest and juice of 1 lime
    (approx. 1 tbsp juice)
1 tbsp fish sauce
1 tbsp sriracha sauce
5g fresh coriander,
    finely chopped

NON-FAST DAY
Serve a double portion,
or add 2–3 tablespoons
cooked brown rice.

Crunchy baby gems filled with sweet, Thai-flavoured pork make an excellent light supper or lunch.

1. Heat the oil in a large wok or frying pan. Add the pork and separate as much as possible with a wooden spoon. Add the lemongrass and stir-fry for 3–4 minutes.

2. Add the ginger, garlic and spring onion, and cook for 1 minute more, stirring all the time. Remove from the heat and set aside to cool slightly.

3. Mix all of the dressing ingredients together in a small bowl or jug. Stir into the pork to coat thoroughly.

4. Serve in baby gem lettuce cups and top with the coriander leaves, if using.

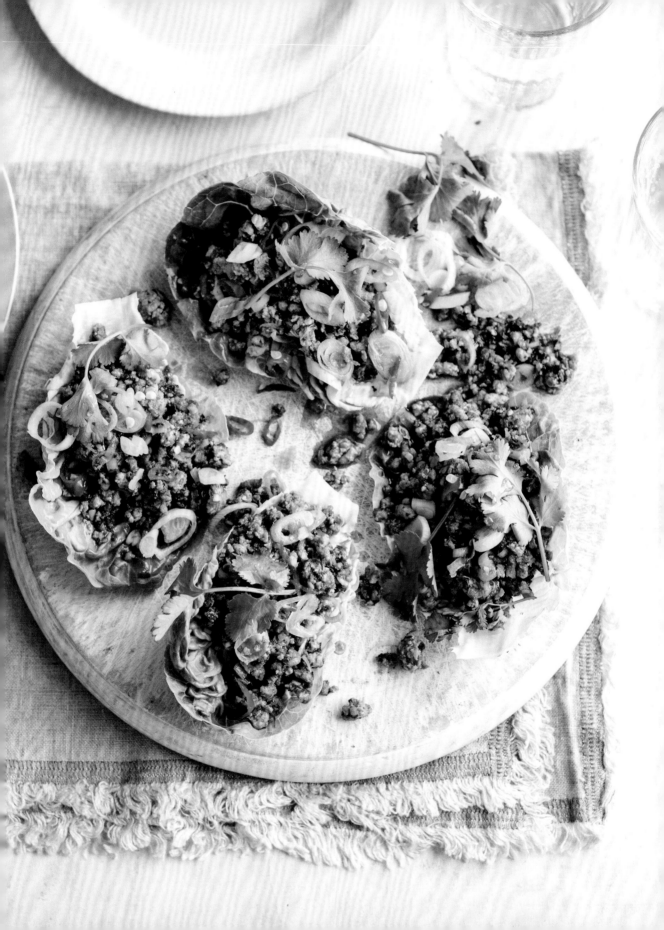

Easy Cauli Steak Pepperoni Pizza

SERVES	PREP	COOK
2	**15** mins	**20** mins

1 large cauliflower
2 tbsp olive oil
3 tbsp tomato purée
2 garlic cloves, peeled
    and finely chopped
1 tsp dried oregano
75g grated mozzarella
30g sliced pepperoni
    or chorizo

COOK'S TIP
You can add or swap in
extra protein – see options
for top-ups on page 240,
such as bacon, diced ham,
diced chicken, extra cheese
or anchovies.

NON-FAST DAY
Have a larger portion –
it's great just as it is!

You don't need to deprive yourself of a good pizza –
this gives you all the flavour with a fraction of the
calories and carbs!

1. Preheat the oven to 190°C/Fan 170°C/Gas 5 and line
a baking tray with baking parchment.

2. Prepare the cauliflower. Cut two slices, 1.5cm thick,
through the centre of the cauliflower, core intact, to create
two whole pieces, or 'steaks'. (Keep the offcuts to make
cauli-rice, which can be frozen for use at another time –
see page 68.)

3. Place the cauliflower steaks on the prepared baking tray
and brush with 1 tablespoon of the olive oil. Roast in the
oven for 10 minutes.

4. Meanwhile, mix the tomato purée, garlic, oregano and
remaining olive oil in a small bowl. Season with a pinch
of salt and plenty of freshly ground black pepper.

5. Remove the cauliflower steaks from the oven and spread
the tomato mixture over them. Scatter the mozzarella all
over and place the pepperoni or chorizo on top. Return
to the oven for a final 10 minutes, or until the cheese is
bubbling and the pepperoni crisp.

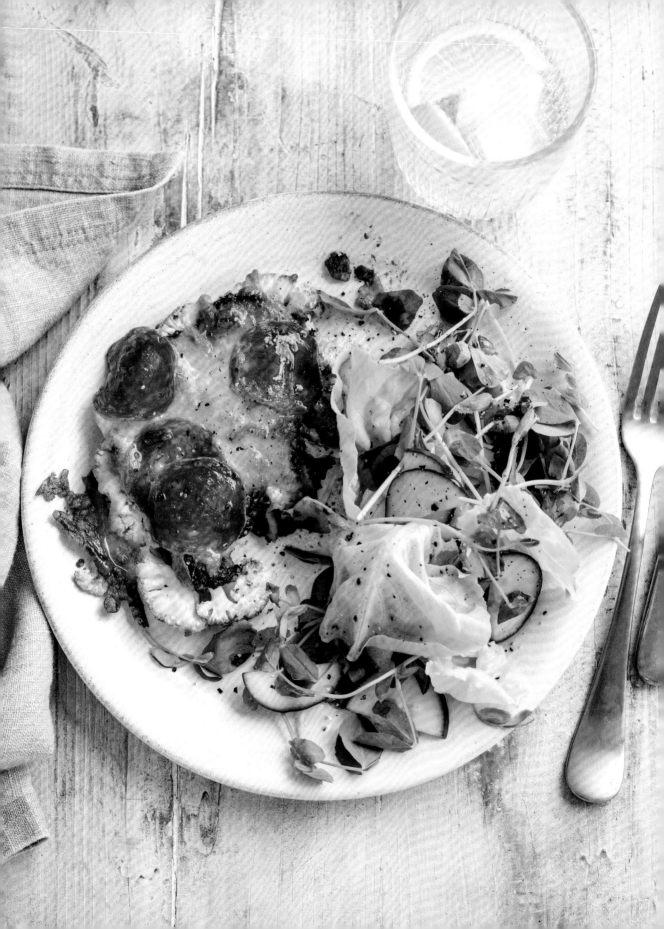

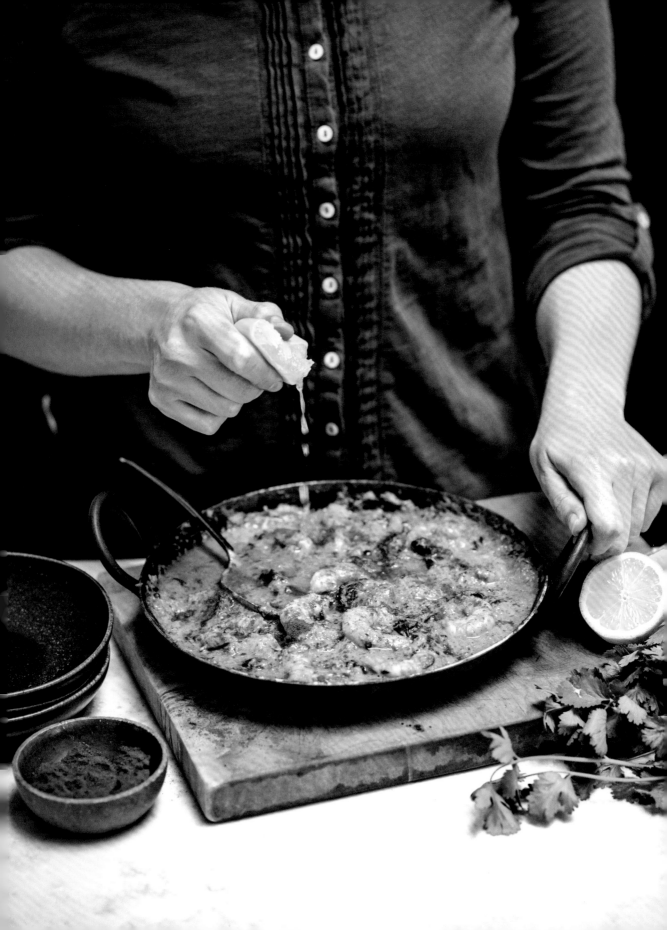

Fish & Seafood

These recipes celebrate the huge variety
of seafood we have on our doorstep.
Fish and seafood are not only delicious,
they are also high in protein and nutrients,
and enable us to top up our often-depleted
yet much-needed reserves of anti-
inflammatory omega-3 oils.

| PER SERVING | **179cals** | PROTEIN **22.6g** | CARBS **3.8g**

Crab Salad with Asian-style Dressing

SERVES	PREP
1	**10** mins

100g green salad leaves

50g cucumber, thinly sliced

5g fresh coriander, leaves picked and left whole

1 portion of Asian Dressing (see page 239)

120g white crab meat (tinned or fresh)

NON-FAST DAY

Double the portion size and add a slice of sourdough to mop up the juices.

I grew up by the sea, regularly cooking and eating crabs and shellfish, and crab remains one of my favourite foods. With its delicate, slightly sweet and slightly salty taste, it's high in protein and nutrients, and the tinned version is highly affordable. We use the white flesh to make a delicious, exotic-flavoured, low-carb salad.

1. Place the salad leaves, cucumber and coriander in a wide-based bowl. Add the dressing and toss to coat.

2. Top with the crab meat and serve.

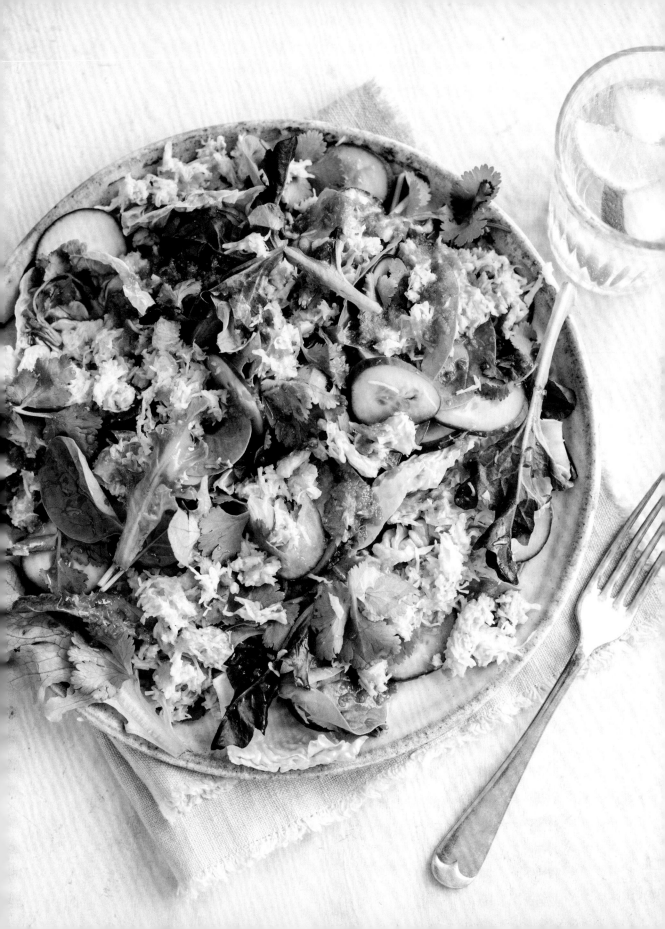

PER SERVING | **438cals** | PROTEIN **30.3g** | CARBS **7.2g**

Roasted Pepper and Cauliflower Tortilla with Prawns and Aioli

SERVES
2

PREP
10
mins

COOK
15
mins

1½ tbsp olive oil
½ small cauliflower (approx.
    250g), cut into slices about
    2mm or as thin as you can
    (include the stalk)
1 roasted red pepper from
    a jar (approx. 70g),
    roughly chopped
½ tsp paprika
150g cooked and peeled prawns
4 medium free-range eggs,
    whisked

For the aioli:
2 tbsp full-fat mayonnaise
2 tbsp full-fat Greek yoghurt
1 tsp garlic granules

NON-FAST DAY
Serve with a few small,
unpeeled baby potatoes.

Spanish tortillas are traditionally made with starchy potato, but this version cleverly substitutes cauliflower, which is super low in carbs and high in nutrients. Serve with a leafy salad.

1. Start by making the aioli – mix the mayo, yoghurt and garlic together in a small bowl and season with salt and freshly ground black pepper.

2. Place the olive oil in a non-stick frying pan over a medium heat, add the cauliflower and fry for 8–10 minutes, until starting to soften and take on some colour.

3. Add the roasted red pepper, paprika and prawns and warm through for 3–4 minutes, stirring occasionally. Pour in the eggs, spread them out evenly and season. Cook for 3–4 minutes, or until the egg is just set.

4. Divide between two plates and top with a spoonful of aioli.

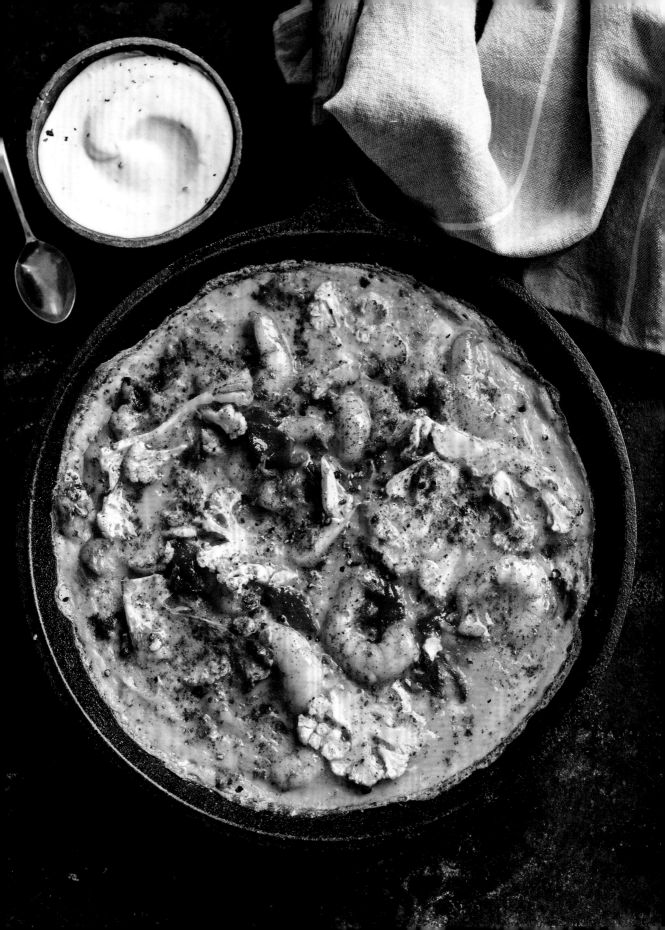

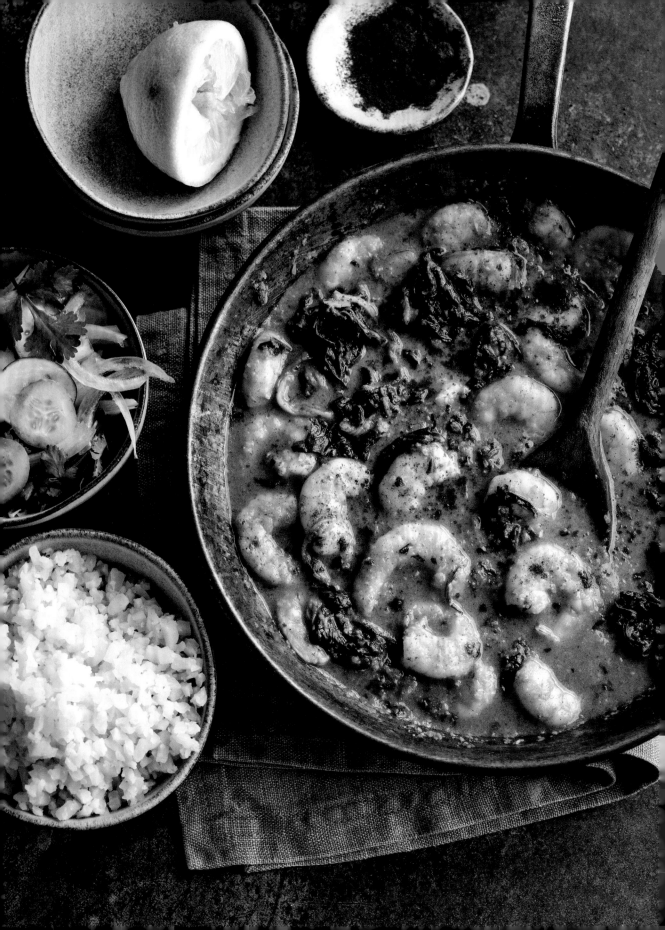

Made-in-Minutes Goan Prawn Curry with Spinach

SERVES | PREP | COOK
4 | **5** mins | **10** mins

1 small leek, trimmed
  and roughly chopped
3 garlic cloves, peeled
20g fresh root ginger
  (no need to peel)
2 tsp ground cumin
1 tsp ground coriander
1 tsp paprika
1 tsp garam masala
1 vegetable stock cube
1 small tomato, quartered
1 tbsp olive oil
1 × 400ml tin full-fat
  coconut milk
100g frozen spinach
400g frozen raw, peeled
  king prawns, defrosted
Juice of ½ lemon (optional)

COOK'S TIP
Get ahead with this recipe
by creating the curry base
up to the point the coconut
milk is added. It will keep
in the fridge for up to 4 days.

NON-FAST DAY
Serve a double portion
and/or serve with 2–3
tablespoons cooked
brown rice.

This luscious dish has the feel of a curry that has been laboured over for hours. The flavour is condensed into a paste, creating the most fabulous, creamy, coconut base for the spinach and prawns. Although it has quite a few ingredients, most are found in the cupboard or freezer. Serve with cauli-rice (see page 68) and steamed leafy greens.

1. Place all the ingredients up to and including the tomato in a food processor and blitz until smooth.

2. Tip the paste into a saucepan, add the oil and fry over a medium heat, stirring from time to time, for 3–4 minutes.

3. Pour in the coconut milk and add the frozen spinach. Simmer for 3–4 minutes to allow the flavours to mingle and the spinach to defrost.

4. Finally, add the defrosted prawns and cook for no more than 2 minutes, until they have just turned pink.

5. Stir through the lemon juice, if using, and serve.

PER SERVING | **502cals** | PROTEIN **41.6g** | CARBS **21.9g**

One Pan Squid Rings with Red Pepper, Feta and Puy Lentils

SERVES | PREP | COOK
2 | **10** mins | **10** mins

1 small onion, peeled and diced

1 medium red pepper, deseeded and sliced

2 tbsp olive oil

125g cooked Puy lentils

140g broccoli florets, any thick stem bases trimmed and sliced lengthwise

300g raw frozen squid rings, defrosted and drained

2 garlic cloves, peeled and finely chopped

100g feta cheese, diced

Pinch of chilli flakes (optional)

2 wedges of lemon, to serve

NON-FAST DAY
Increase the portion size and add a generous drizzle of olive oil.

A super-tasty one-pan dish, based on the classic combination of Puy lentils, sweet red peppers and tangy feta. Puy lentils are much loved by your gut microbiome, thanks to the fibre, which also boosts weight loss. You could serve this with a nice crunchy salad.

1. Place the onion, red pepper and oil in a large frying pan over a medium heat and sweat for 3–4 minutes.

2. Stir in the lentils, broccoli and squid and cook for 5 minutes, stirring occasionally. Add the garlic in the last minute.

3. Scatter over the feta, season with freshly ground black pepper and sprinkle in the chilli flakes, if using. Add 2–3 tablespoons of water and cover with a lid or some foil. Reduce the heat and cook gently for about 3 minutes, until the broccoli is cooked.

4. Serve with lemon wedges.

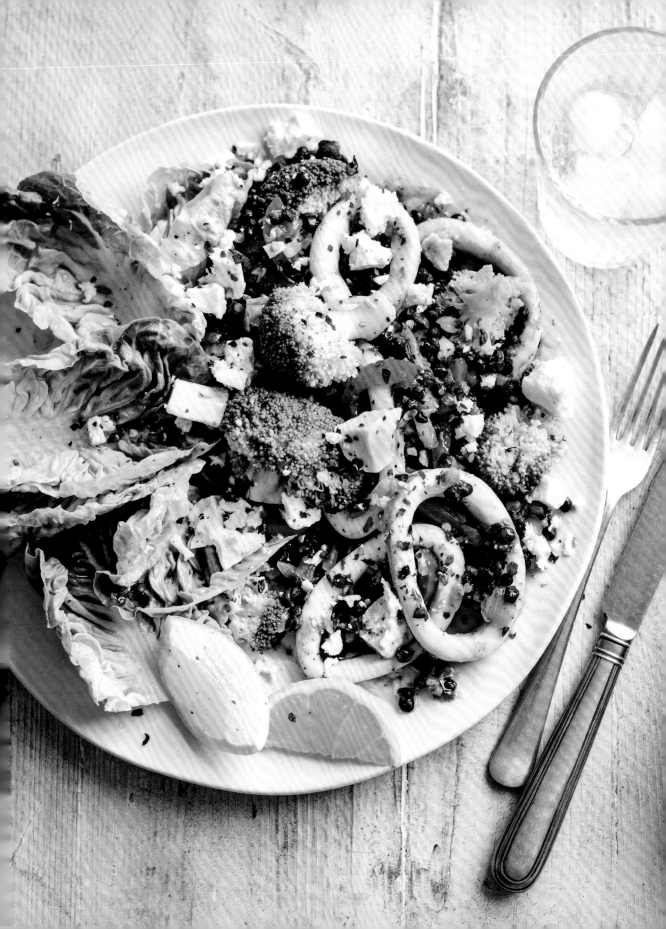

PER SERVING | **236cals** | PROTEIN **25g** | CARBS **4.4g**

White Fish with Herby Green Dressing and Lentils

SERVES | PREP | COOK
2 | **5** mins | **5** mins

2 white fish fillets (such as cod, hake or basa), defrosted if frozen (approx. 240g total weight)
½ tbsp olive oil
3 tbsp cooked beluga or Puy lentils from a pack, warmed through

For the herby green dressing:
1½ tbsp olive oil
1 sprig of rosemary (optional), leaves picked
20g fresh parsley
20g fresh dill
3 anchovy fillets
1 tbsp cider vinegar

NON-FAST DAY
Increase the portion size and/or serve with 2–3 tablespoons wholegrains or unpeeled baby potatoes with butter or olive oil.

The zingy dressing here transforms the fish, which is a blessing for people, like Michael, who are not natural fish eaters but enjoy it if there is plenty of added flavour. Serve with leafy greens or a colourful salad.

1. Fry the fish in the olive oil over a medium heat for 4–5 minutes, turning halfway.

2. Place all the dressing ingredients in a bowl or jug and blitz with a stick blender. Add a splash of water to loosen – it should be the consistency of pesto.

3. Spoon the herby green dressing over the fish and serve with the lentils and some steamed green veg.

Keto Fish Pie

SERVES	PREP	COOK
4	**15** mins	**30–40** mins

1 large cauliflower, broken into 2cm florets and stalk roughly chopped (approx. 700g prepared weight)

2½ tbsp olive oil

1 medium onion, peeled and finely chopped

350g fish pie mix (e.g. salmon, smoked haddock and cod)

200ml full-fat milk

150g full-fat cream cheese

10g fresh dill or parsley, roughly chopped (or 1 tsp dried)

50g Cheddar, grated

NON-FAST DAY
Increase the portion size and scatter with toasted seeds or chopped nuts.

A scrumptious keto take on a classic fish pie, with no hint of the usual stodgy ingredients of potato and flour. This luxurious alternative uses roasted cauliflower in place of the mash and creamed cauliflower to thicken the sauce, proving that you can still enjoy flavourful comfort food! Serve with French beans or broccoli.

1. Preheat the oven to 220°C/Fan 200°C/Gas 8.

2. Place 150g of the cauliflower in a food processor and blitz until fine. Place the remaining cauliflower in a baking dish measuring 28 × 20cm and toss with 1½ tablespoons of the olive oil. Season with salt and freshly ground black pepper and roast in the oven for 25 minutes, stirring halfway through.

3. Meanwhile, place the onion and remaining oil in a saucepan and sauté over a medium heat for 3–4 minutes. Remove the onion from the pan and set aside. Add the fish to the pan and cover with the milk. Slowly bring to the boil, then simmer gently for 2 minutes.

4. Remove the fish with a slotted spoon and set aside. Add the cream cheese to the pan with the milk and whisk until combined. Then add the blitzed cauliflower and cooked onions to this creamy mixture and simmer for 2 minutes. Remove from the heat, stir in the fish and dill or parsley and check the seasoning.

5. Remove the cauliflower from the oven and preheat the grill to high. Remove the cauliflower from the baking dish and set aside. Pour the fish mixture into the dish, then top with the roasted cauliflower. Scatter over the Cheddar and place under the grill for 5 minutes, or until the cheese is bubbling and golden.

PER SERVING | **366cals** | PROTEIN **27.5g** | CARBS **3.9g**

Southern Prawn Patties with Ranch Dressing

SERVES **2** | PREP **10–15** mins | COOK **5–7** mins

For the Prawn Patties:
½ small red onion, peeled and roughly chopped
1 garlic clove, peeled and roughly chopped
½–1 tsp chilli flakes, to taste
4 level tbsp ground almonds (approx. 40g)
Zest of 1 lemon
1 medium free-range egg
10g fresh coriander
225g cooked and peeled prawns, drained
1 tbsp olive oil

For the Ranch Dressing:
2 tbsp full-fat Greek yoghurt
1 tbsp full-fat mayonnaise
½ tsp garlic granules
1 tsp lemon juice

NON-FAST DAY
Have a larger portion.

Inspired by a southern Mississippi recipe for shrimp, this recipe has bold flavours of prawn, garlic and chilli and a tangy dressing. Serve with a large, crunchy salad.

1. Place the onion, garlic, chilli flakes, ground almonds, lemon zest, egg and three-quarters of the coriander in a bowl and blitz with a stick blender, or in a food processor, until finely chopped. Add the prawns and blitz briefly, leaving some texture. Season generously with salt and freshly ground black pepper.

2. Transfer the mixture to a plate and shape it into 4 burger-size patties, about 2.5cm thick. Refrigerate for 30 minutes for best results.

3. Meanwhile, combine all the dressing ingredients with the remaining coriander in a small bowl. Mix well and season.

4. Place the olive oil in a non-stick frying pan over a medium heat. Fry the patties on each side for 3 minutes, until hot through and starting to crisp. Serve with the Ranch Dressing alongside.

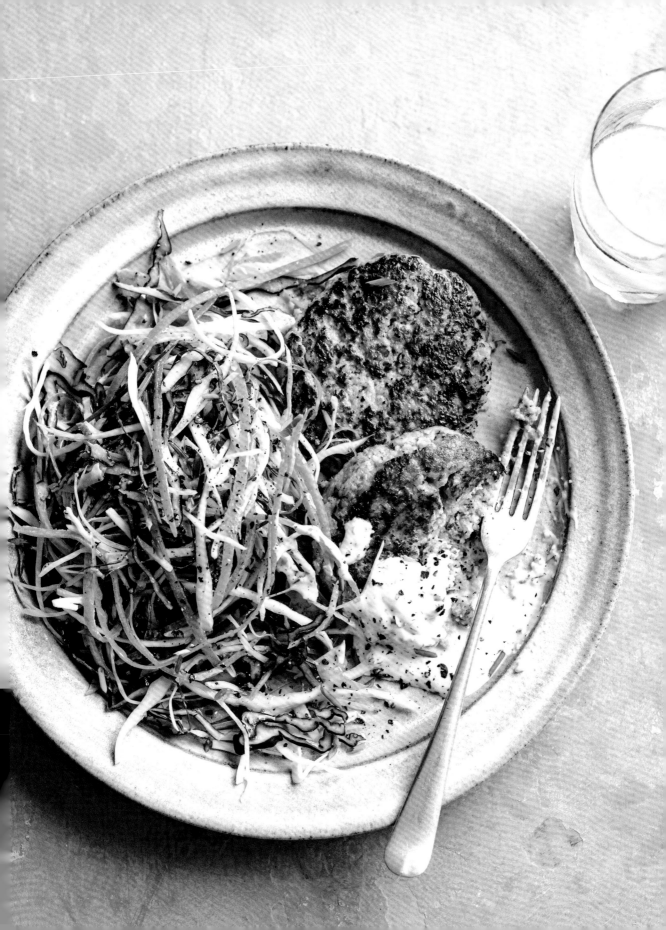

PER SERVING | **486cals** | PROTEIN **30.6g** | CARBS **10.5g**

Scallops with a Mushroom and Sun-dried Tomato Sauce

SERVES | PREP | COOK
2 | **5** mins | **5–7** mins

240g frozen scallops,
   defrosted
1 tbsp olive oil
2 sun-dried tomatoes from
   a jar, finely chopped,
   plus 1 tbsp of the oil
100g chestnut mushrooms,
   finely sliced
1 large garlic clove (or 2
   small cloves), peeled
   and finely chopped
100ml crème fraîche
5g fresh dill, roughly chopped

NON-FAST DAY
Have a larger portion
and add some cooked
peas or beans.

This recipe is super quick to make and results in a truly restaurant-level meal. I use frozen scallops as they are cheaper and readily available in supermarkets. Serve with a generous plate of greens.

1. Season the scallops with a pinch of salt and freshly ground black pepper. Place the oil in a non-stick frying pan over a high heat. When it is really hot, add the scallops and fry on one side for 2 minutes, until they have a golden crust. Turn and fry on the other side for 1 minute, then remove from the pan and keep warm.

2. Add the sun-dried tomato oil to the pan with the mushrooms and sauté for 1 minute.

3. Stir in the garlic and sun-dried tomatoes and fry for 30 seconds.

4. Add the crème fraîche, dill and 1 tablespoon of water to loosen. Stir to heat through and return the scallops to the pan for a final 30 seconds. Check the seasoning and serve.

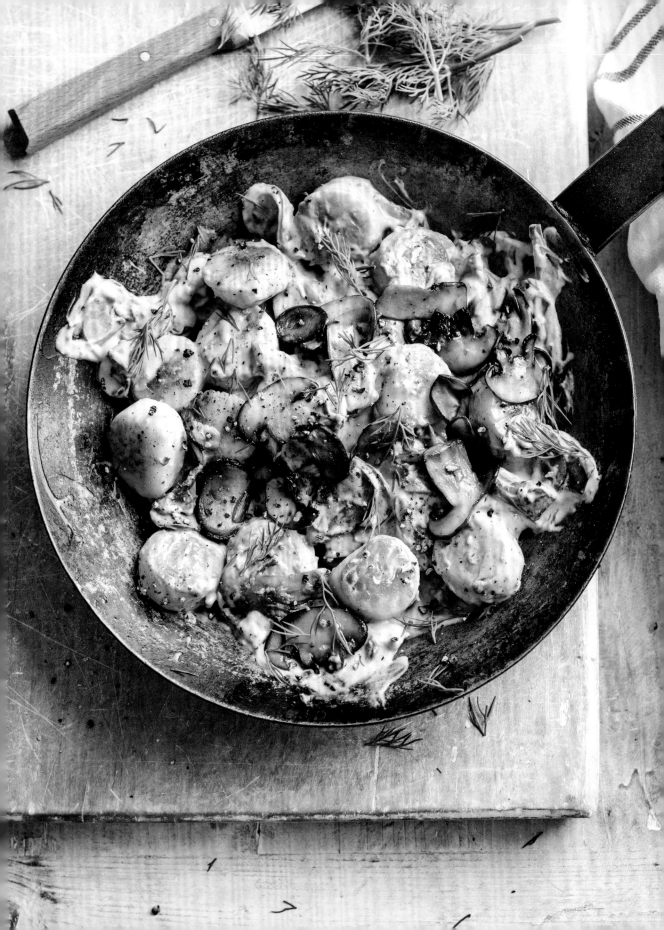

Diced Salmon, Ginger and Veg Bowl

SERVES
2

PREP
15–20
mins

200g white cabbage,
thinly sliced
1 medium red pepper,
deseeded and finely diced
1 small ripe avocado, peeled,
stone removed and
roughly chopped
2 cooked salmon fillets
(approx. 90g each)
1 tbsp sesame seeds
2 tsp soy sauce

For the dressing:
2 tsp sesame oil
1 tsp olive oil
1 tbsp cider vinegar
1 ball stem ginger from a jar,
finely chopped
Pinch of chilli flakes (optional)

NON-FAST DAY
Increase the portion size and
serve with 2–3 tablespoons
cooked quinoa or brown rice.

Throw-together food for when you really don't feel like cooking. With its subtle flavours of sesame, ginger and soy, this South-East-Asian-inspired bowl will leave you feeling satisfied yet full of energy.

1. Firstly, make the dressing. Combine all the ingredients in a small bowl or jug, season with salt and lots of freshly ground black pepper and mix well.

2. Divide the cabbage, red pepper, avocado and salmon between two wide bowls. Drizzle the dressing all over and gently toss to coat. Finish with the sesame seeds and soy sauce, and serve immediately.

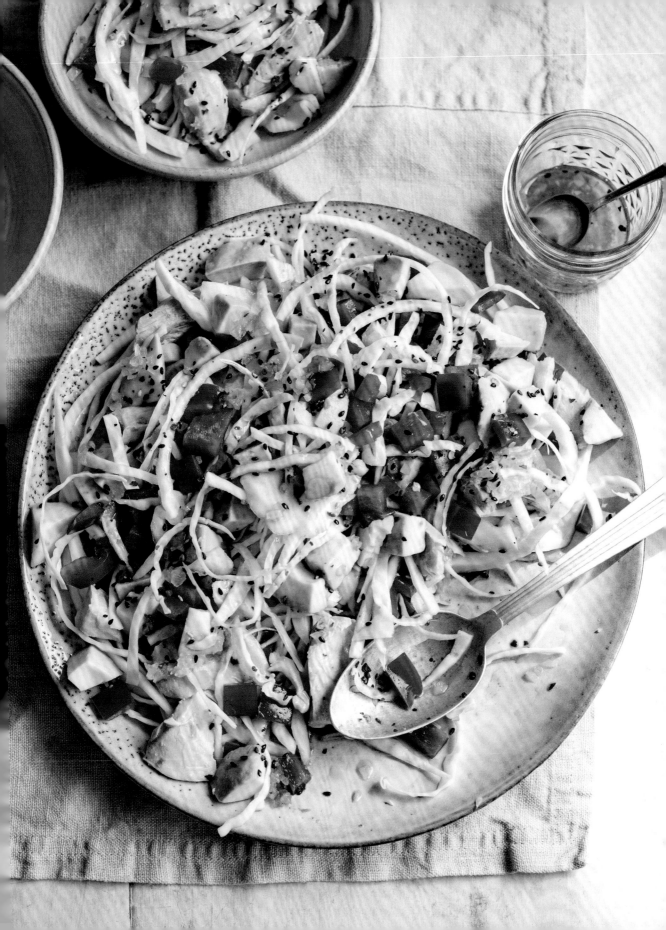

Spicy Salmon and Butternut Squash Traybake

SERVES	PREP	COOK
2	**20** mins	**25** mins

½ onion, peeled and sliced into thin wedges about 1cm thick
200g butternut squash, peeled and cut into 1.5cm dice
1 medium red pepper, deseeded and sliced
1 tsp medium curry powder
1 tbsp olive oil
¼ × tin full-fat coconut milk
1 large garlic clove, peeled and finely chopped
1 tsp fresh root ginger, peeled and finely chopped
2 salmon fillets (approx. 130g each)
2 tbsp Thai fish sauce

NON-FAST DAY
Enjoy a larger portion and/or serve with 2–3 tablespoons cooked wholegrain rice.

We all love traybakes – throw in the ingredients, let the oven do its bit and, hey, presto! Here the mildly curried veg contrasts with the salmon in its creamy, spiced coconut sauce.

1. Preheat the oven to 200°C/Fan 180°C/Gas 6.

2. Place the onion, squash and red pepper in a medium baking dish and sprinkle the curry powder over the top. Drizzle with the olive oil and toss to combine. Roast in the oven for 15 minutes.

3. Remove from the oven and gently stir in the coconut milk, garlic and ginger. Place the salmon on top, drizzle with the fish sauce and season with salt and freshly ground black pepper. Return to the oven for 10 minutes, or until the salmon is cooked through.

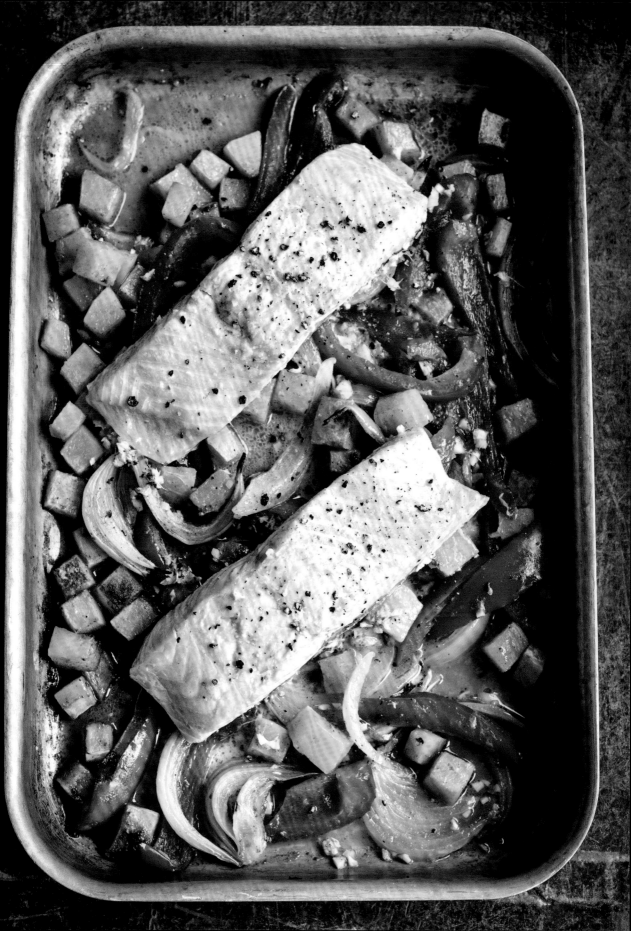

PER SERVING | **259cals** | PROTEIN **17.2g** | CARBS **3.4g**

Salmon, Ginger and Coriander Fish Cakes with Soy and Lime

SERVES	PREP	COOK
2	**15** mins	**4** mins

150g salmon fillet,
  skin removed
10g fresh root ginger,
  peeled and finely grated
5g fresh coriander,
  finely chopped
1 level tbsp ground almonds
1 tbsp olive oil
2 tbsp soy sauce
Juice of ½ lime (approx. 1 tbsp)

NON-FAST DAY
Increase the portion
size and/or serve with
wholegrain noodles
or 2–3 tablespoons
cooked wholegrain rice.

Fresh and clean in flavour – without a starchy coating – these fish cakes need little more than some lettuce leaves on the side (peppery rocket works well) to make a great lunch. A generous plate of steamed greens will make them into a delicious dinner.

1. Place the salmon on a clean work surface and, using a very sharp knife, chop finely. The salmon should be slightly paste-like, but still have small chunks.

2. Transfer the salmon to a bowl and add the ginger, coriander and ground almonds. Season generously with salt and freshly ground black pepper and mix until thoroughly combined. Shape into four small patties, squeezing each one between the palm of your hands to make sure it is tightly packed together.

3. Heat the olive oil in a non-stick frying pan over a medium heat and fry the fish cakes for 2 minutes on each side. Transfer to a sheet of kitchen roll to mop up the excess oil.

4. Meanwhile, mix the soy sauce and lime juice together in a dipping bowl and serve alongside the fish cakes.

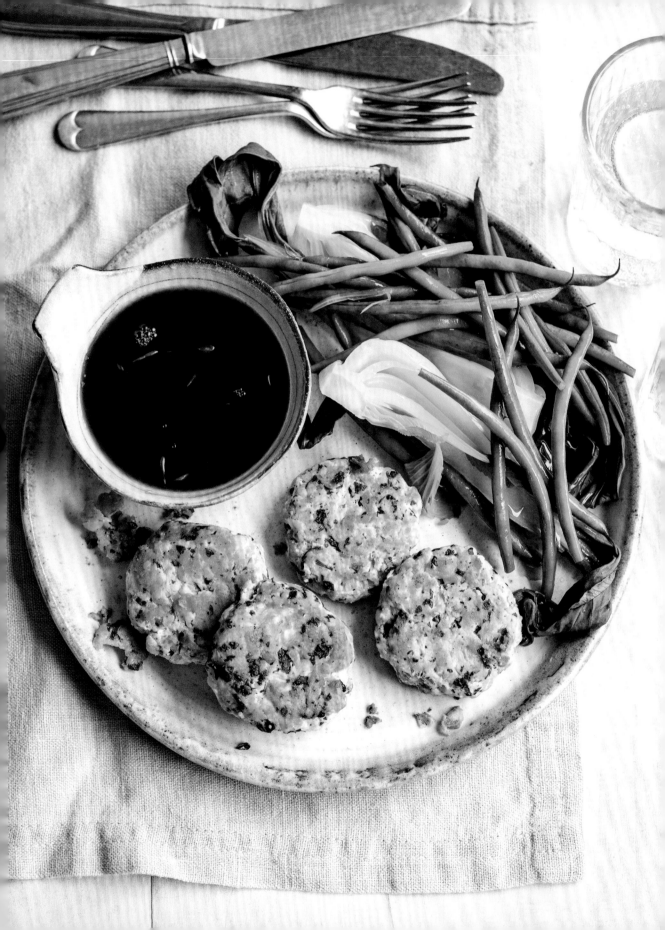

PER SERVING | **494cals** | PROTEIN **30.9g** | CARBS **18.5g**

Beetroot Tzatziki with Roasted Aubergine and Baked Salmon

SERVES **2** | PREP **15** mins | COOK **30** mins

1 aubergine, cut into
   2cm pieces
2 tbsp olive oil
½ tsp cumin seeds
½ small cauliflower,
   broken into 2cm florets
150g cooked beetroot,
   drained and chopped
1 garlic clove, peeled and
   finely chopped
3 tbsp full-fat Greek yoghurt
1 tbsp cider vinegar
10g fresh mint, leaves picked
   and roughly chopped
50g rocket
2 pre-cooked salmon or
   smoked mackerel fillets,
   skin removed, roughly flaked
   (approx. 170g total weight)
½ tsp ras-el-hanout (optional)
1 tbsp mixed seeds
¼ lemon, for squeezing

NON-FAST DAY
Enjoy a larger portion
and serve with a
wholemeal pitta.

This is a vibrant dish bursting with colour, texture and flavour, and deserves to be celebrated on a platter!

1. Preheat the oven to 200°C/Fan 180°C/Gas 6.

2. Spread the aubergine on one side of a large baking tray and drizzle with 1 tablespoon of the oil. Add the cumin seeds, season with salt and freshly ground black pepper and toss together. Bake in the oven for 10 minutes.

3. Meanwhile, toss the cauliflower with the remaining oil and some salt and pepper. Remove the tray from the oven and spread the cauliflower out beside the aubergine. Return to the oven for another 20 minutes, until the vegetables are soft and nicely browned.

4. Remove the tray from the oven, cover the aubergine to keep warm, and transfer the cauliflower to a large bowl or jug, along with the beetroot, garlic, yoghurt and cider vinegar. Blitz with a stick blender until smooth. Stir in the mint, reserving a few leaves to garnish, and season to taste.

5. Spread the purple tzatziki on a platter, top with the rocket, roasted aubergine and salmon or mackerel fillets. Sprinkle with the ras-el-hanout, if using, a scattering of seeds and a squeeze of lemon juice to serve.

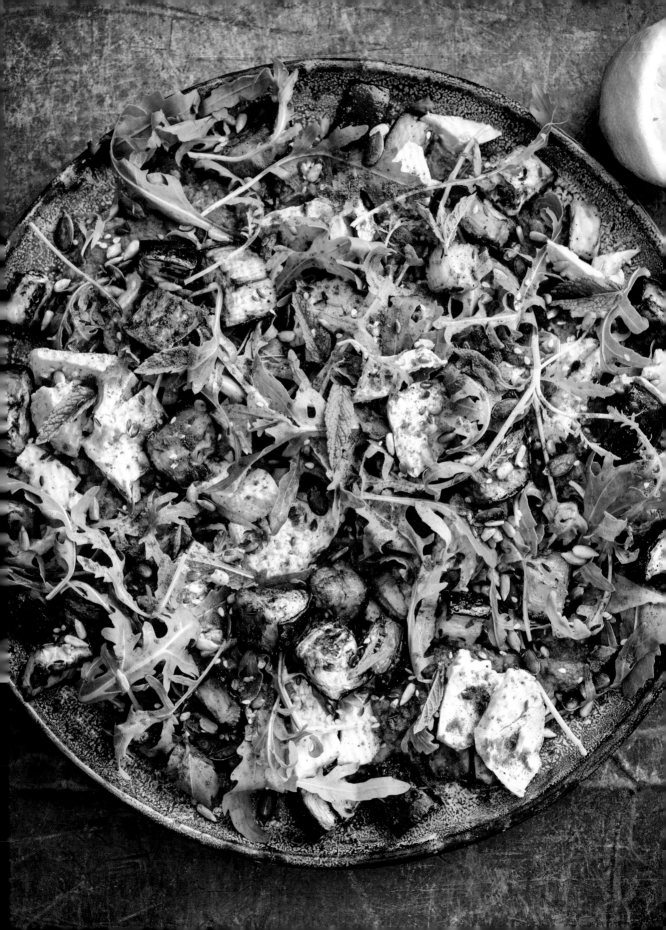

PER SERVING | **215cals** | PROTEIN **32.2g** | CARBS **6.5g**

Diced Miso Tuna with Spinach and Quinoa

SERVES | PREP | COOK
2 | **10** mins | **3–4** mins

1 tsp sesame oil
1 tsp soy sauce
2 tsp white miso paste
Zest of ½ lime and juice
   of 1 lime
¼ tsp chilli flakes (optional)
2 tuna steaks (approx. 240g
   total weight), cut into
   1cm dice
½ tbsp olive oil
200g fresh spinach
2 heaped tbsp cooked
   quinoa (approx. 35g)

NON-FAST DAY
Increase the portion size.

If you are not keen on fish, this recipe will surely convert you. And it's a seriously good source of protein.

1. Combine the sesame oil, soy sauce, miso paste, lime zest, half the lime juice and the chilli flakes, if using, in a bowl. Stir in the tuna and toss to coat.

2. Place a large frying pan over a medium heat and add the olive oil and spinach. Gently wilt the spinach, stirring from time to time, then add the quinoa to heat through.

3. Transfer the spinach and quinoa to two warmed plates and return the pan to the heat. Increase the heat, add the tuna and cook for about 1 minute, tossing it once or twice, but leaving it pink in places.

4. Divide between the two plates and drizzle with the remaining lime juice to serve.

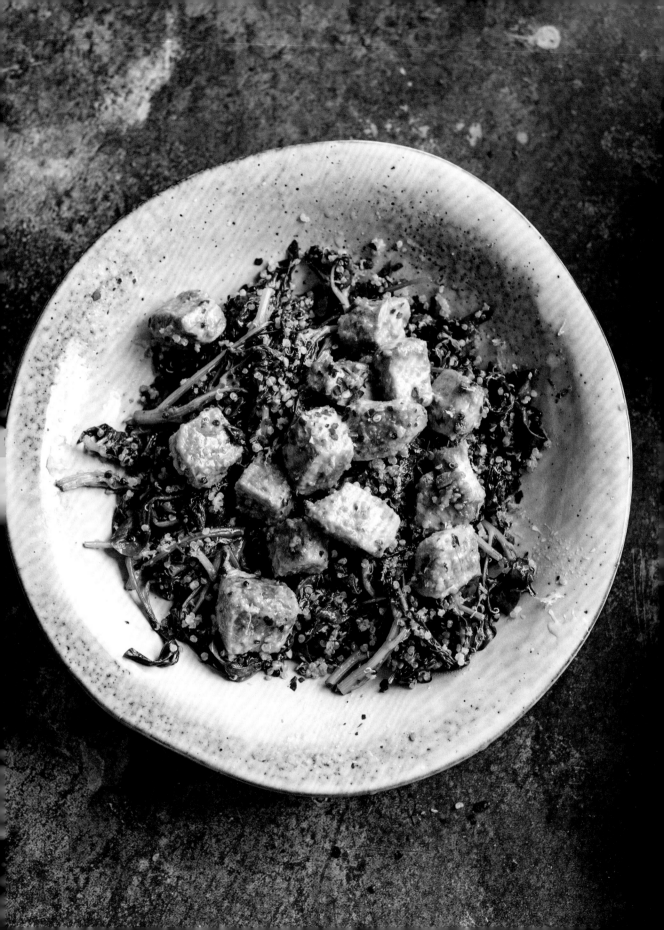

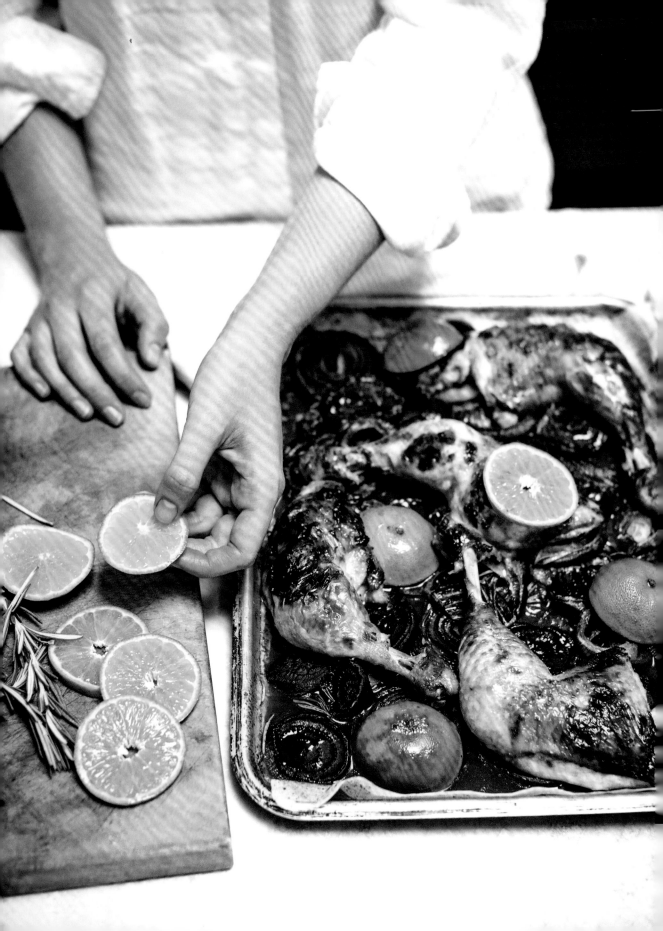

Chicken, Turkey & Duck

Asian Duck with Beansprout Noodles,
Piri Piri Roast Chicken with Jalapeño
Yoghurt, casseroles, burgers, traybakes,
stir-fries... This chapter offers tasty,
healthy protein every which way.

PER SERVING | **255cals** | PROTEIN **34.3g** | CARBS **13.8g**

Spicy Korean Chicken Bowl with Kimchi and Cauliflower Rice

SERVES **2** | PREP **15–20** mins | COOK **4** mins

A comforting bowl packed with flavour and easy to make. Great for a lunchbox, too. Kimchi is a Korean dish made of spicy fermented vegetables and is available to buy in most supermarkets.

2 boneless, skinless chicken thighs, chopped into 1cm chunks (approx. 250g total weight)
1 tbsp soy sauce
2 garlic cloves, peeled and finely grated
Juice of ½ lime
1 tbsp sriracha sauce
300g cauli-rice (see page 68)
1 pak choi, leaves separated and finely sliced
50g frozen edamame beans, defrosted
50g kimchi
1 portion Sriracha Yoghurt Dressing (see page 236)

NON-FAST DAY
Serve a double portion and/or add some wholegrain noodles.

1. Place the chicken, soy sauce, garlic, lime juice and sriracha sauce in a bowl and mix well. Leave to marinate for 30 minutes, if time allows.

2. Fry the chicken in a wok or frying pan over a medium heat for 3–4 minutes, or until cooked through and the sauce has thickened and coats the chicken.

3. Divide the cauli-rice, pak choi, edamame beans, kimchi and chicken between two bowls. Drizzle with the Sriracha Yoghurt Dressing and serve.

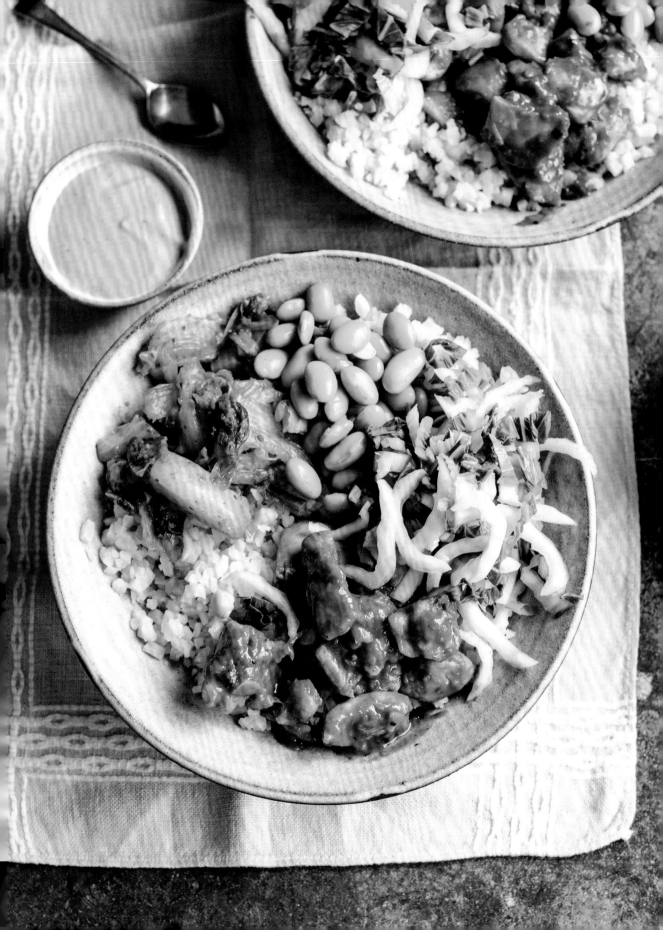

Keto-fried Chicken

SERVES	PREP	COOK
2	**10** mins	**12** mins

80g ground almonds
½ tsp flaked sea salt
1 tsp freshly ground
   black pepper
½ tsp cayenne pepper
1 egg
4 large skinless, boneless
   chicken thighs (approx.
   400g total weight), each
   cut into three
1 tbsp olive oil

NON-FAST DAY
Have a bigger portion and/or
serve with 2–3 tablespoons
cooked wholegrain rice.

Crispy, delicious and packing a real punch with the
pepper and cayenne seasoning, these nuggets will be
your go-to keto-fried chicken, supplying most of your
daily protein, yet only 2.6g carbs. Serve with the
Simple Coleslaw (see page 193).

1. Preheat the oven to 200°C/Fan 180°C/Gas 6.

2. Combine the ground almonds, salt, black and cayenne
pepper in a bowl. Crack the egg into a separate bowl
and whisk.

3. Dip each piece of chicken in the egg, then the ground
almond mixture until thoroughly coated.

4. Heat the oil in a large frying pan over a medium heat
and fry the chicken pieces for 1 minute on each side,
until golden. Transfer to a baking tray and roast in
the oven for 10 minutes, until cooked through.

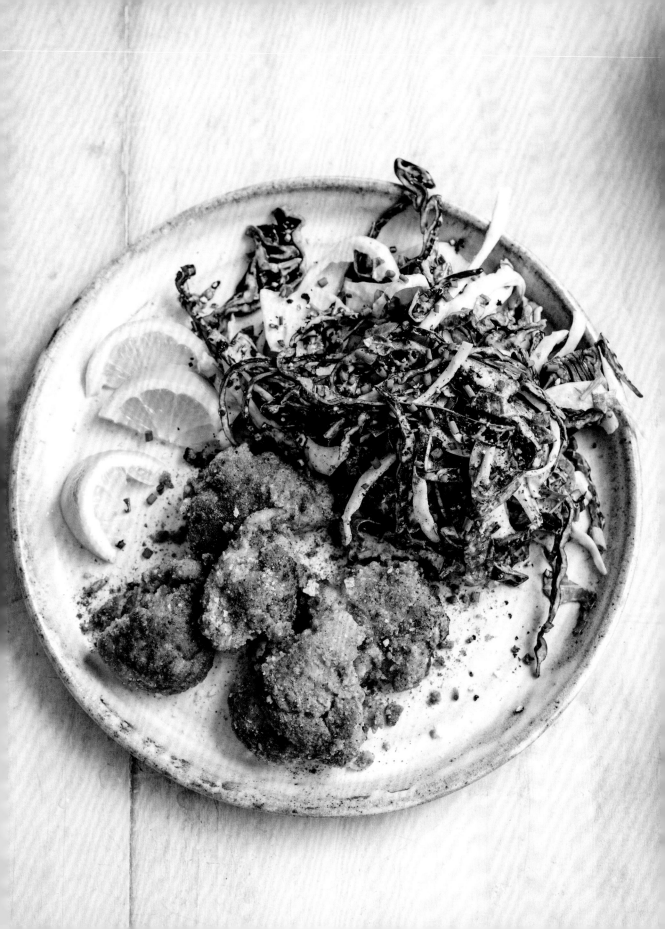

PER SERVING | **210cals** | PROTEIN **27.4g** | CARBS **3.9g**

Baked Tandoori Chicken with Garlic Raita

SERVES	PREP	COOK
4	**25** mins	**30** mins

80g tandoori paste
80g full-fat Greek yoghurt
10–15g fresh root ginger,
    peeled and diced
4 skinless bone-in chicken
    thighs (approx. 450g
    total weight)

For the garlic raita:
2 tbsp full-fat Greek yoghurt
1 small garlic clove, peeled
    and finely chopped
¼ cucumber or ½
    courgette, grated
¼ tsp cumin seeds (optional)

NON-FAST DAY
Have a double portion,
and/or serve with
2–3 tablespoons
cooked brown rice.

A fabulously flavourful combination. With enough for four portions, Michael and I ate half of it with dahl and cauli-rice one night, and had the remaining two portions the following day with a generous, dressed salad (see pages 236–9 for no-count dressings).

1. Mix the tandoori paste, yoghurt and ginger in a large bowl. Add the chicken and mix to coat well. Marinate for 30–60 minutes, if time allows.

2. Preheat the oven to 200°C/Fan 180°C/Gas 6 and line a baking tray with baking parchment.

3. Place the chicken on the prepared baking tray and roast in the oven for about 25 minutes, turning halfway, or until cooked through.

4. Meanwhile, to make the raita, stir the yoghurt, garlic and cucumber or courgette together in a small bowl and season with salt and freshly ground black pepper. Scatter with the cumin seeds, if using.

5. Serve the tandoori chicken, hot or cold, with the raita and your choice of steamed greens or salad.

Chicken Traybake with Beetroot and Orange

SERVES | **PREP** | **COOK**
2 | **45** mins | **35** mins

Zest and juice of 1 lemon
1 tsp Dijon mustard
2 tsp sweet chilli sauce
2 chicken legs, skin on,
   excess fat trimmed
   (approx. 500g total weight)
1 red onion, peeled and sliced
125g cooked beetroot, sliced
2 sprigs of rosemary, leaves
   picked, or ½ tsp dried
1 tbsp olive oil
2 tangerines, unpeeled,
   1 sliced in half horizontally,
   1 sliced in rings

NON-FAST DAY
Serve with 2–3 tablespoons
wholegrain rice, quinoa or
bulgur wheat and dress with
an extra drizzle of virgin
olive oil.

This recipe is adapted from a fabulous meal made by old friends. Tangy, sweet and juicy, it is low in carbs and delivers really well on the protein front. Serve with half a plate of steamed greens.

1. Mix the lemon zest and juice, Dijon mustard, sweet chilli sauce and a generous pinch of salt and some freshly ground black pepper in a bowl. Add the chicken and toss to coat. Set aside to marinate for 30 minutes.

2. Preheat the oven to 200°C/Fan 180°C/Gas 6 and line a baking tray with baking parchment.

3. Place the onion, beetroot and rosemary on the prepared tray and drizzle with the oil. Arrange the chicken legs on top and pour the marinade all over. Dot the tangerine halves cut-side-down around the chicken legs and roast everything in the oven for 20 minutes.

4. Remove the tray from the oven and place the tangerine rings on top of the chicken. Return to the oven and roast for a further 15 minutes, until the chicken is golden and the onion silky soft.

5. Allow the dish to cool slightly before squeezing the juice from the halved tangerines into the sauce. Check the seasoning and serve.

Piri Piri Roast Chicken with Jalapeño Yoghurt

SERVES
4

PREP
10–12
mins

COOK
90
mins

1 roasted red pepper
  from a jar (approx. 70g)
1 tbsp piri piri seasoning
2 tbsp olive oil
1 tbsp soy sauce
1 × 1.5kg whole chicken,
  at room temperature
1 lemon, pierced a few times
  with a fork (optional)

For the jalapeño yoghurt:
30g jalapeños from a jar,
  drained
125g full-fat Greek yoghurt
10g fresh coriander

NON-FAST DAY
Increase the portion
size and/or serve with
2–3 tablespoons cooked
quinoa, wholegrain rice,
bulgur wheat or roasted
butternut squash.

How to transform the humble roast chicken so it sings with flavour... If making for less than four, simply strip the leftover meat from the bone, store in the fridge and keep as a base for another quick and easy meal. Serve with a generous portion of greens.

1. Preheat the oven to 200°C/Fan 180°C/Gas 6.

2. Place the roasted red pepper, piri piri seasoning, olive oil and soy sauce in a small jug and blitz with a stick blender until smooth. Season with freshly ground black pepper.

3. Pull the skin away from the crown of the chicken, creating a pocket between the flesh and the skin. Add half the piri piri mixture and spread out under the skin. Pour the rest over the chicken and rub in. Place the lemon in the cavity of the chicken, if using, season once more and place in a roasting tin. Cover with foil and roast in the oven for 1 hour 10 minutes. Remove the foil and roast for a final 20 minutes.

4. Meanwhile, prepare the jalapeño yoghurt. Place all the ingredients in a small jug and blitz with a stick blender until smooth. Season.

5. Divide the chicken between four plates and serve the jalapeño yoghurt alongside.

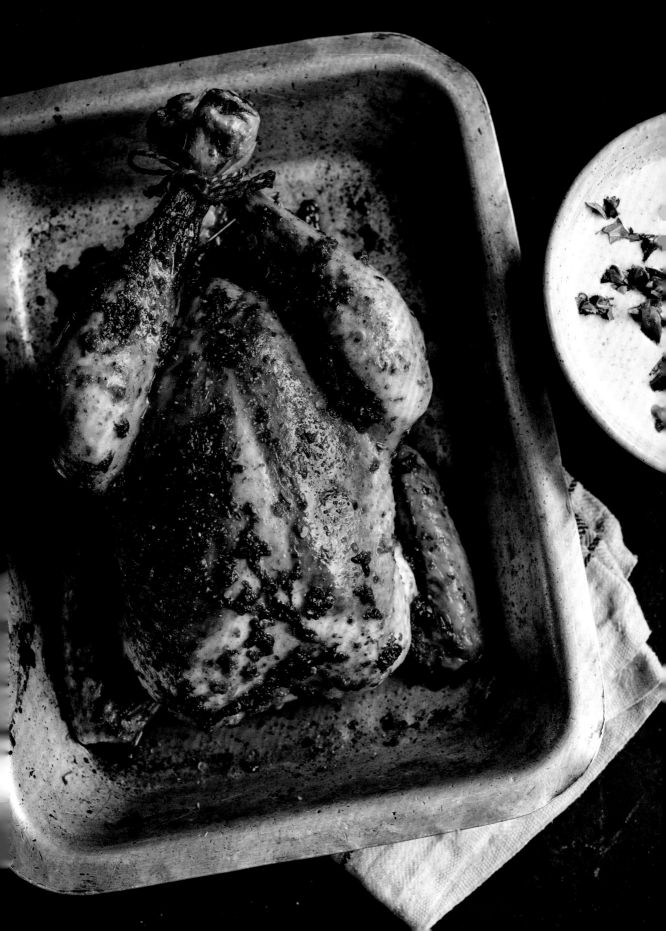

PER SERVING | **281cals** | PROTEIN **45.1g** | CARBS **3g**

Red Pepper, Sun-dried Tomato and Feta Stuffed Chicken

SERVES | PREP | COOK
4 | **15–20** mins | **25** mins

1 roasted red pepper from a jar, finely chopped (approx. 70g)
1½ tbsp sun-dried tomato pesto
80g feta cheese, crumbled
4 chicken breast fillets (approx. 165g each)
½ tbsp olive oil
240g tenderstem broccoli

COOK'S TIP
These stuffed chicken breasts keep well in the fridge for a day or two once cooked and make a great addition to a salad for a quick lunch.

A tasty dish suitable for all the family with plenty of protein to keep you feeling full for longer.

1. Preheat the oven to 200°C/Fan 180°C/Gas 6 and line a baking tray with baking parchment.

2. Place the roasted red pepper, pesto and feta cheese in a bowl and mix until thoroughly combined. Season with a pinch of salt and freshly ground black pepper.

3. Place each chicken breast between two pieces of baking parchment and use a rolling pin to flatten slightly, ensuring they are an even width. Using a very sharp knife, cut a deep slit down the length of each breast. Spoon a quarter of the feta mixture into each pocket and press it down firmly. Place each breast on the baking tray, drizzle with the olive oil, season again and bake in the oven for 25 minutes.

4. Just before the chicken is ready, quickly steam or boil the broccoli. Serve the chicken with the broccoli and drizzle some of the juices from the tray all over.

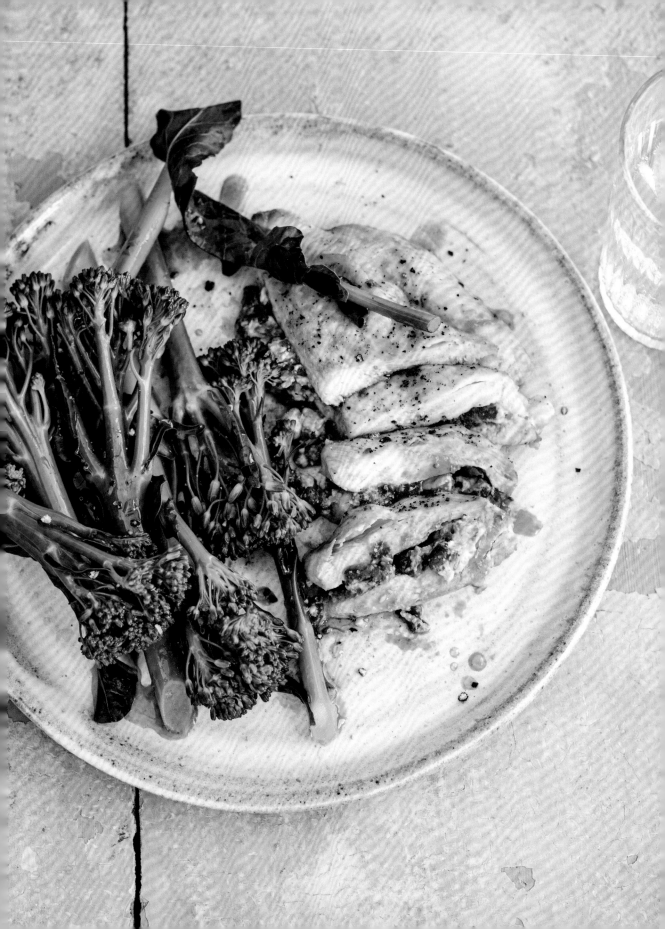

Hummus-crusted Chicken and Savoy Cabbage Traybake

SERVES **2** | **PREP** **10** mins | **COOK** **30** mins

2 tbsp hummus (approx. 50g)
½ tsp paprika, plus a little extra to dust
2 chicken breast fillets (approx. 300g total weight)
½ savoy cabbage, stalk and any large ribs discarded, leaves cut into 1cm slices
2 garlic cloves, peeled and finely chopped
2 tbsp olive oil
2 wedges of lemon
2 tsp nigella seeds (optional)

COOK'S TIP
You could try different flavours of hummus. Alternatively, it's easy to make your own.

NON-FAST DAY
Serve with 2–3 tablespoons bulgur wheat or brown rice and some peas or beans.

This is a great way to use up leftover hummus (the coarser the hummus the better the crust). The fibre in the hummus supports a healthy gut microbiome, which in turn contributes to better immunity, reduced inflammation and improved mood. Win-win! Serve with half a plate of leafy veg or salad.

1. Preheat the oven to 200°C/Fan 180°C/Gas 6 and line a large baking tray with baking parchment.

2. Mix the hummus with the paprika and spread evenly over the chicken breasts. Dust with a little extra paprika, season with salt and freshly ground black pepper and roast in the oven for 15 minutes.

3. Remove the tray from the oven and scatter the cabbage and garlic around the chicken. Drizzle with the oil, season and toss gently. Return to the oven for a further 15 minutes.

4. To serve, divide between two plates and squeeze the lemon juice all over. Finish with a scattering of nigella seeds, if using.

Chicken Casserole with Chorizo, Thyme and Olives

SERVES
4

PREP
15–20
mins

COOK
40
mins

(plus an optional 30 minutes to marinate)

4 skin-on, bone-in chicken thighs, trimmed (approx. 750g total weight)
Juice of 1 lemon
2 tbsp olive oil
1 large onion, peeled and thinly sliced
50g chorizo, diced
1 whole garlic bulb, top stem removed, cloves unpeeled, sliced horizontally into two halves
1 × 400g tin small white beans (such as cannellini), drained
100g pitted green olives, halved
½ tsp dried thyme or 5–6 sprigs of fresh thyme
200g tenderstem broccoli, any thick stems trimmed and split lengthways

NON-FAST DAY
Serve with 2–3 tablespoons cooked pearl barley or wholegrain rice and drizzle with an extra glug of olive oil.

This is great one-pot keto comfort food, using a whole bulb of garlic, which turns sweet and fragrant on cooking. Garlic also has numerous health benefits and antioxidant properties. It's said to improve blood pressure and reduce 'bad' cholesterol, and even reduce the risk of heart disease and dementia.

1. If time permits, marinate the chicken in the lemon juice for 30 minutes prior to cooking. Preheat the oven to 190°C/Fan 160°C/Gas 5.

2. Place a heavy-based casserole (with a fitted lid) over a medium heat and fry the chicken, skin-side-down, in 1½ tablespoons of the olive oil until browned. This should take about 4 minutes. Reserve the lemon juice if the chicken has been marinating.

3. Turn over to seal on the other side for 30 seconds, then push the thighs to one side of the pan or transfer to a bowl while you cook the onions and chorizo. Fry for 2 minutes until slightly softened. Return the chicken to the middle of the pan and add the halved garlic bulb. Drizzle the remaining oil over the garlic. Pour in the reserved lemon juice, along with 200ml water. Stir in the beans, olives and thyme, add a generous pinch of salt and freshly ground black pepper, cover with the lid and place in the oven for 25 minutes.

4. Remove from the oven and squeeze the softened garlic from its skin (tongs are useful for this). Use a fork to roughly mash the garlic into the juices. Place the broccoli on top of the chicken, cover with the lid and return to the oven for a final 10 minutes.

Bang Bang Chicken

SERVES	PREP	COOK
4	**5** mins	**40** mins

4 small chicken legs
  (approx. 250kg each)
2 tbsp soy sauce
1 heaped tbsp crunchy peanut
  butter (no added sugar)
2 balls stem ginger from
  a jar, finely chopped
  (approx. 40g total weight)
1 tsp chilli flakes (to taste)
1 tsp sesame oil
2 tbsp olive oil

NON-FAST DAY
Serve with a few
tablespoons brown rice
and scatter with roughly
chopped toasted peanuts.

Sweet spicy chicken legs are a family favourite.
Here they are sweetened by stem ginger in syrup.
Some pak choi braised in one teaspoon of sesame
oil (one small bulb per person, sliced into quarters
lengthways) would go well with it, as would other
sliced leafy greens – no need to count the calories.

1. In a large bowl, toss the chicken legs in the soy sauce.
If time permits, marinate for 30 minutes, or longer.

2. Preheat the oven to 200°C/Fan 180°C/Gas 6 and line
a baking tray with baking parchment.

3. Place the chicken legs on the prepared tray and roast
in the oven for 20 minutes.

4. Meanwhile, mix the remaining ingredients together
in a small bowl. Add water to loosen, if necessary.

5. Remove the chicken from the oven and cover with
the sauce. Return to the oven for a final 20 minutes,
or until cooked through.

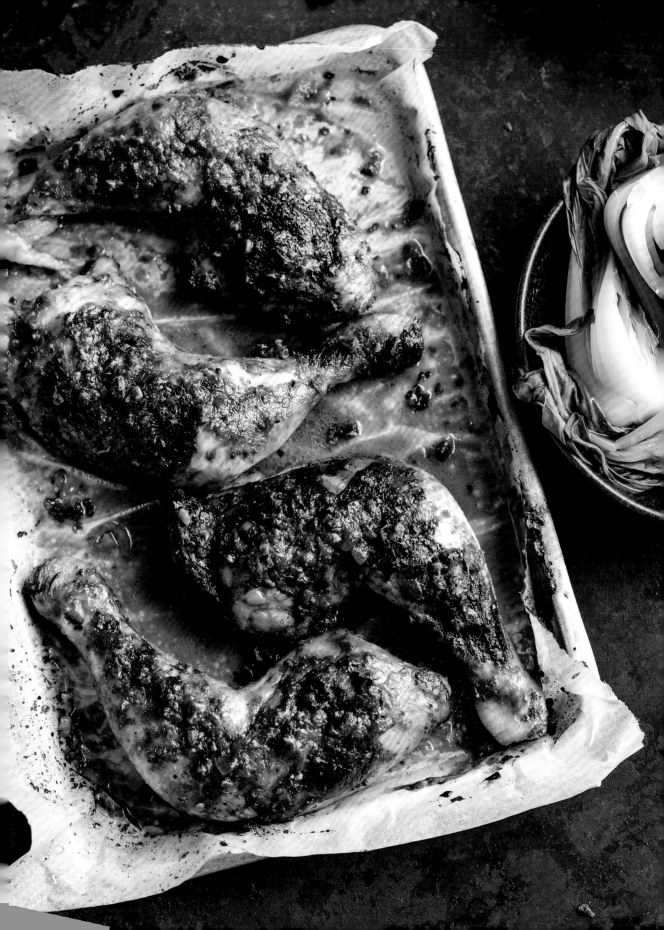

PER SERVING | **383cals** | PROTEIN **43.9g** | CARBS **11.5g**

Chicken and Fennel Traybake with Roasted Garlic and Parsley Sauce

SERVES	PREP	COOK
2	**10** mins	**40** mins

1 large fennel bulb, trimmed,
  halved lengthwise and
  sliced, reserving some
  fronds to garnish
1 red pepper, deseeded
  and sliced
2 tbsp olive oil
3–4 sprigs of thyme,
  leaves picked (or ½ tsp
  dried thyme)
1 tsp dried tarragon (optional)
Juice of 2 lemons
  (approx. 4 tbsp)
2 chicken breast fillets,
  flattened if thick
  (approx. 150g each)
1 bulb of garlic, top
  stem removed
10g Parmesan, finely grated
2 tbsp full-fat Greek yoghurt
5g fresh flat-leaf parsley,
  roughly chopped

NON-FAST DAY
Increase your portion
size and/or serve with
2–3 tablespoons cooked
quinoa, wholegrain rice
or pearl barley, and a
drizzle of olive oil.

Roasted garlic sweetens beautifully in the oven, and for this simple traybake it is mixed into a creamy dressing. Serve with plenty of colourful or green non-starchy veg.

1. Preheat the oven to 200°C/Fan 180°C/Gas 6.

2. Place the fennel and red pepper in a medium baking dish and drizzle with 1 tablespoon of the olive oil. Season with a generous pinch of salt and freshly ground black pepper. Roast in the oven for 10 minutes.

3. Remove the tray from the oven and mix in the herbs and lemon juice. Place the chicken on top of the veg and place the garlic cut-side-up alongside. Drizzle the remaining oil over the garlic and chicken and return to the oven for 25–30 minutes, or until the chicken juices are running clear. Remove from the oven and set aside to rest.

4. Carefully squeeze the soft roasted garlic from the bulb and place in a small bowl along with the Parmesan, yoghurt and parsley. Mix well, season and drizzle over the chicken. Sprinkle with the reserved fennel fronds to serve.

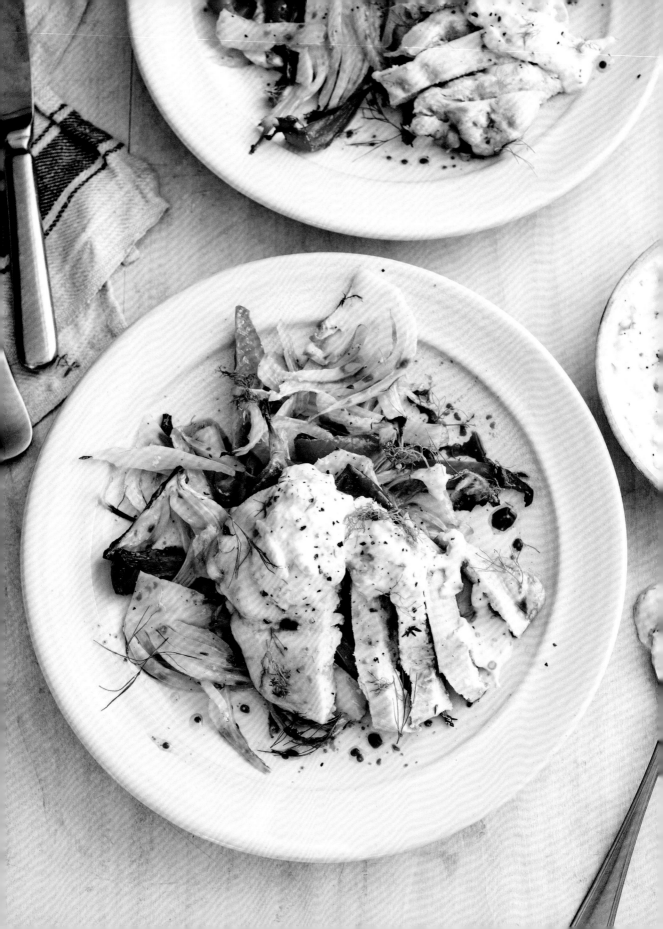

Mozzarella Chicken

SERVES	PREP	COOK
2	**10** mins	**35** mins

2 tbsp olive oil
½ onion, peeled and diced
2 garlic cloves, peeled and finely sliced
1 × 400g tin chopped tomatoes
Small handful fresh basil, roughly chopped, some leaves kept whole to garnish
200ml vegetable stock
250g skinless chicken breast
60g fresh mozzarella, sliced

Of the hundreds of recipes in the Fast 800 Online Programme, this one, with its golden cheesy topping, has been one of the most popular. So, we are sharing it with you, too. Serve with a crunchy green salad or any non-starchy vegetables.

1. Preheat the oven to 190°C/Fan 170°C/Gas 5.

2. Place the oil, onion and garlic in a frying pan over a medium heat and sauté for 5 minutes, or until the onion softens.

3. Add the chopped tomatoes, chopped basil and stock then bring to the boil. Reduce the heat and leave to simmer and thicken for 5 minutes, stirring occasionally.

4. Meanwhile, place the chicken breast between two sheets of parchment paper and use a rolling pin or something heavy to lightly pound it to increase the surface area. Place the chicken in an ovenproof dish, cover it with the tomato sauce and place the slices of mozzarella on top. Roast in the oven for about 20 minutes, or until the chicken is completely cooked through and the cheese is melted and golden.

5. Sprinkle with the remaining basil leaves to serve.

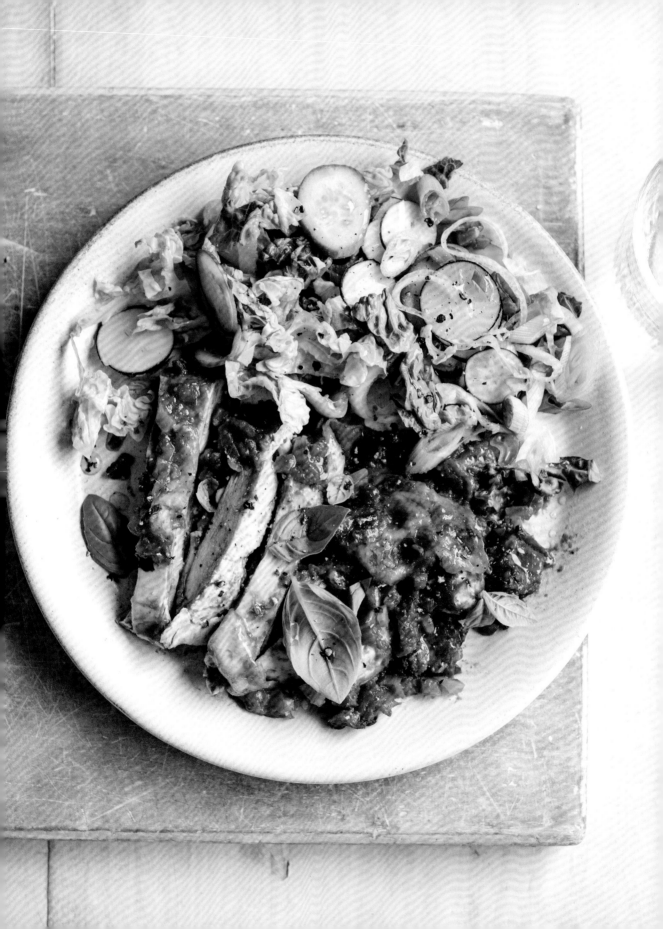

PER SERVING | **267cals** | PROTEIN **38.5g** | CARBS **9.1g**

Ginger and Orange Stir-fried Chicken

SERVES	PREP	COOK
2	**5** mins	**8–10** mins

2 tbsp oyster sauce

Zest of ½ orange and
   1 tbsp of juice

20g fresh root ginger,
   peeled and finely chopped

1 tbsp olive oil

2 chicken breast fillets
   (approx. 300g total weight),
   very finely sliced

1 × 300g shop-bought vegetable
   stir-fry pack, preferably
   without baby corn

NON-FAST DAY

Increase the portion size
and/or serve with wholemeal
noodles or 2–3 tablespoons
wholegrain rice.

This super-quick and easy recipe will beat any takeaway stir-fry. It is also low-carb, promotes ketosis and helps to shed the pounds. Slice the chicken as thinly as you can, as this will help it cook more quickly and retain its moisture. Serve with cauli-rice (see page 68).

1. Mix the oyster sauce, orange zest, juice and ginger together in a small bowl and set aside.

2. Place the oil in a wok or heavy-based frying pan over a high heat. When smoking hot, add the chicken and stir-fry for 4 minutes. Remove the chicken from the pan and set aside.

3. Add the vegetables to the pan with a generous splash of water – this will create lots of steam, which helps the veg cook quickly. Stir-fry for 3–4 minutes, adding a splash more water, if necessary.

4. Return the chicken to the pan and pour in the sauce. Cook for 2 minutes until thoroughly heated through.

Duck Breasts with Rocket, Mustard and Puy Lentils

SERVES **2**

PREP **5–7** mins

COOK **35** mins

1 tbsp olive oil
½ small onion, peeled
  and finely chopped
2 sticks celery, finely chopped
2 garlic cloves, peeled
  and chopped
½ tsp dried thyme (or 4 sprigs
  of thyme, leaves picked)
50g dried Puy lentils
400ml chicken stock
2 duck breasts, skin scored
  (approx. 170g each)
1 tbsp Dijon mustard
40g rocket

COOK'S TIP
If you don't have an
ovenproof frying pan,
simply transfer the duck
to a baking tray before
placing in the oven.
If you can't find duck
breasts, chicken legs
would work, too. They
take 35–40 minutes at
the same oven temperature.

NON-FAST DAY
Add more Puy lentils.

Duck is a fabulously juicy and highly nutritious meat, which, with the mustardy lentils here, makes a truly harmonious flavour combination. By frying the duck skin-side-down in a hot pan first, you render out the fat and crisp up the skin.

1. Preheat the oven to 200°C/Fan 180°C/Gas 4.

2. Place the oil, onion, celery, garlic and thyme in a medium saucepan, cover with a lid and sauté for 5 minutes, stirring a couple of times.

3. Add the lentils and stock, bring to a gentle simmer and cook, covered, for 30 minutes.

4. Meanwhile, prepare the duck. Pat the duck breasts dry and season the skin with salt and freshly ground black pepper. Place an ovenproof frying pan over a high heat. When hot, place the duck in the pan skin-side-down and fry for 5 minutes, until the skin is crisp and golden – it will smoke a little. Turn the breasts and seal on the other side for 1 minute. Transfer to the oven for 8–10 minutes (medium rare–medium). Remove from the oven and set aside to rest for 5 minutes.

5. Gently stir the Dijon mustard into the lentils, followed by the rocket, just before serving alongside the duck.

PER SERVING | **460cals** | PROTEIN **48.8g** | CARBS **20.3g**

Asian Duck with Bean Sprout Noodles

SERVES	PREP	COOK
2	**15** mins	**20** mins

2 duck breasts
   (approx. 170g each)
1 medium onion, peeled
   and finely chopped
1 tsp garam masala
½–1 tsp chilli powder
50g dried apricots,
   roughly chopped
200ml chicken stock
   (made using
   ½ stock cube)
150g bean sprouts
100g fresh spinach

NON-FAST DAY
Enjoy a larger portion
and/or serve with
2–3 tablespoons cooked
wholegrain rice, quinoa
or wholegrain noodles.

The fruity, tangy and mildly curried sauce contrasts superbly with the richness of the duck in this recipe. Serve the sliced duck on top of cooked greens or on a nest of mixed veg for colour and crunch.

1. Preheat the oven to 200°C/Fan 180°C/Gas 6.

2. Pat the duck breasts dry, then score the skin with a sharp knife and season with salt and freshly ground black pepper.

3. Place a frying pan over a high heat and, when hot, place the duck skin-side-down in the pan. Fry for 5 minutes, until the skin is crisp and golden – it will smoke a little, so it's worth putting on the extraction fan. Turn the breasts and seal on the other side for 1 minute. Transfer to a baking tray, reserving the fat in the frying pan, and roast in the oven for 8–10 minutes for medium rare–medium (still pink in the middle). Set aside to rest for 5 minutes.

4. Meanwhile, place the frying pan back over a medium heat and fry the onion for 3–4 minutes, until softened. Add the garam masala, chilli powder, apricots and stock and simmer for 2 minutes. Pour into a jug and blitz with a stick blender until smooth. Check seasoning.

5. Place the bean sprouts and spinach on a baking tray and pour in the sauce. Cook in the oven for 2–3 minutes, until warmed through and the spinach is wilted. Carefully slice the duck and serve on top of a pile of the veg.

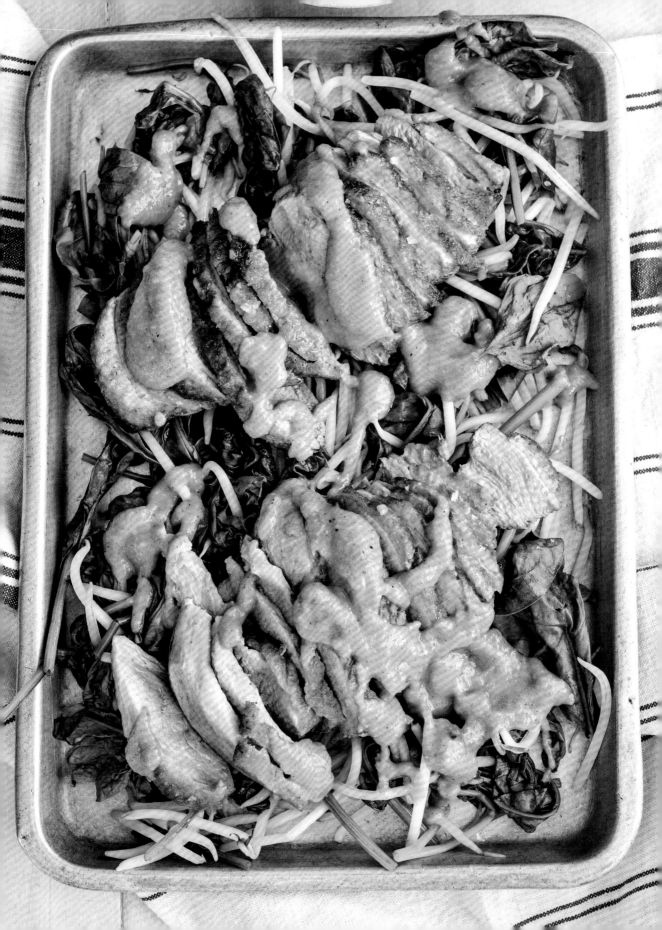

Greek Turkey Burgers with Harissa Yoghurt

SERVES **4** | **PREP** **15** mins | **COOK** **25** mins

½ medium red onion, peeled and finely chopped
40g pitted black olives, finely chopped
50g feta cheese, crumbled
40g Cheddar, grated
1½ tsp dried oregano
500g turkey thigh mince
1 tbsp olive oil
1 level tbsp harissa paste
4 tbsp full-fat Greek yoghurt
1 head of romaine lettuce, leaves separated
2 medium tomatoes, sliced

NON-FAST DAY
Increase the portion size and/or serve with cooked quinoa, bulgur wheat or Instant Mug Bread (see page 206).

You'll love these burgers that are bursting with delicious Mediterranean flavours. If you don't have harissa, sun-dried tomato pesto works well, too. Serve with a generous green salad. You could munch these burgers between two robust lettuce leaves, or see page 205 for a keto bun.

1. Preheat the oven to 200°C/Fan 180°C/Gas 6 and line a baking tray with baking parchment.

2. Place the onion, olives, cheeses, oregano, turkey mince, ½ tablespoon of the olive oil and a generous pinch of salt and freshly ground black pepper in a bowl. Use your hands to thoroughly mix everything together.

3. Shape the mixture into four burgers and place on the baking tray. Drizzle the remaining olive oil all over and roast in the oven for 25 minutes.

4. Meanwhile, mix the harissa and yoghurt together in a small bowl.

5. When the burgers are ready, allow to cool slightly then serve with a couple of lettuce leaves per person and a few slices of tomato. Spoon the cooking juices over the burgers and top with a generous dollop of harissa yoghurt.

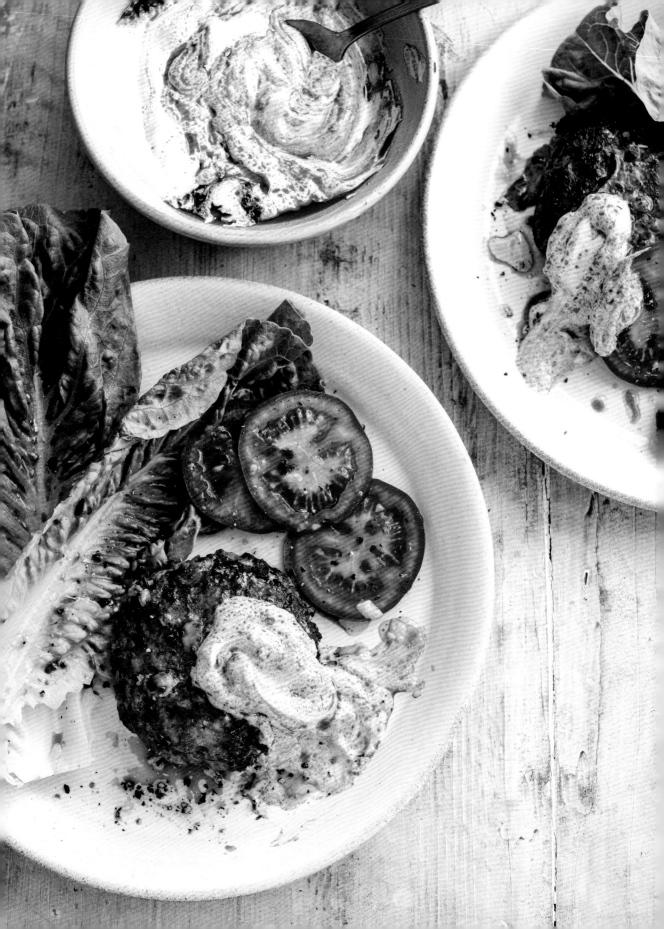

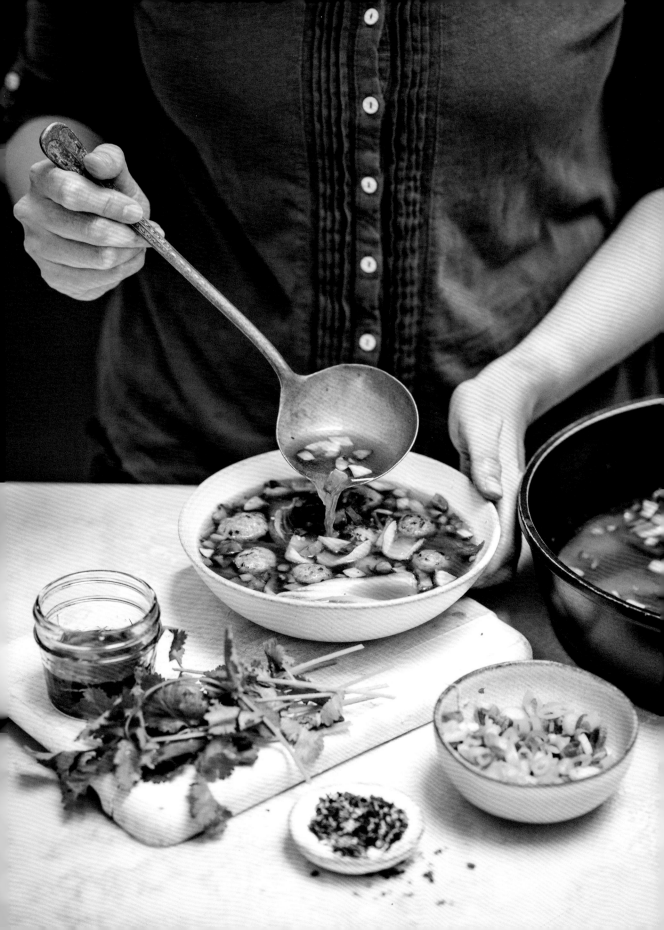

Pork, Lamb & Beef

Meat is a great source of high-quality protein, and you will find some tempting winners here – Steak with Romesco Sauce, Easy Sausage Traybake and a melt-in-the-mouth Cheesy Fajita Beef Casserole... Who says a keto diet can't offer comfort food?

Michael's Mediterranean Stir-fry

SERVES **2** | **PREP** **10** mins | **COOK** **5** mins

1 small head of broccoli,
  cut into small florets
  and stalks diced
½ medium onion,
  peeled and diced
30g chorizo, diced
2 tbsp olive oil
4 tbsp cold, cooked quinoa
  or bulgur wheat
2 garlic cloves, peeled
  and finely chopped
8 cherry tomatoes, halved
100g feta cheese, diced
  or crumbled
Pinch of chilli flakes (optional)

NON-FAST DAY
Enjoy a bigger portion and
drizzle with extra olive oil.

An (almost) one-pan meal, featuring Michael's favourite secret ingredient chorizo, with its warm, smoky flavour that can transform just about anything.

1. Place the broccoli in a large pan of boiling water and cook for 2 minutes. Drain well, reserving some of the cooking water.

2. Place the onion, chorizo and oil in a frying pan over a medium heat and fry for 3–4 minutes, until the onion is softened.

3. Add the quinoa, drained broccoli, garlic and tomatoes and heat through. Add 1 tablespoon of the broccoli cooking water, to loosen.

4. Scatter the feta over the top and season with plenty of freshly ground black pepper and a pinch of chilli flakes, if using.

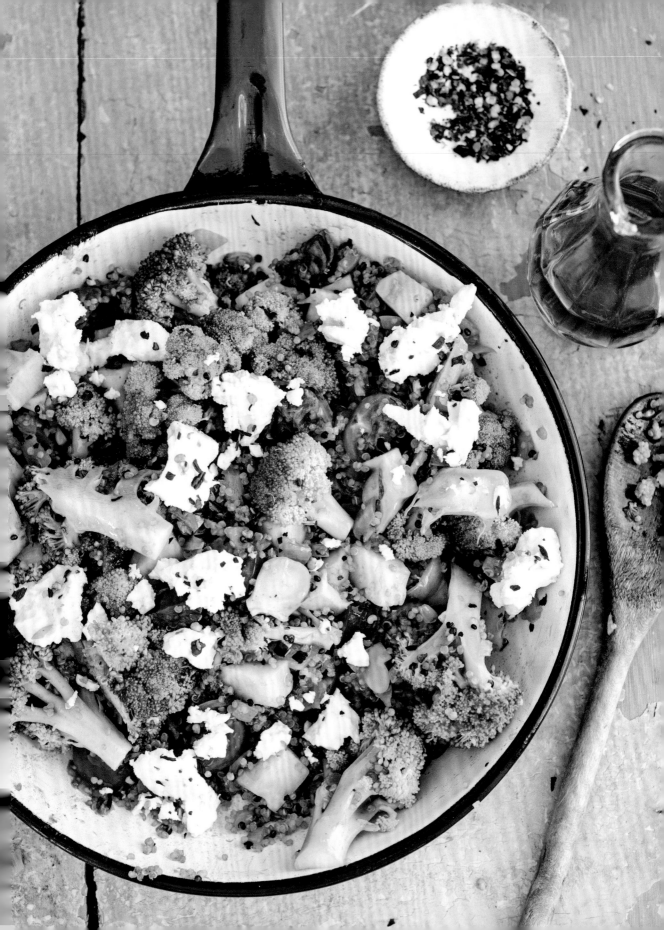

| PER SERVING | **308cals** | PROTEIN **28.6g** | CARBS **7.5g**

Chinese Pork Balls in Mushroom Miso Broth

SERVES | PREP | COOK
2 | **10–15** mins | **15** mins

250g pork mince
15g fresh root ginger, peeled
    and coarsely grated
1 tsp chilli flakes
5g fresh coriander,
    finely chopped
2 tsp sesame oil

For the broth:
100g chestnut mushrooms,
    finely chopped
1 tsp olive oil
2 tbsp white miso
2 tbsp soy sauce
1 pak choi, leaves
    roughly chopped
1 spring onion,
    finely chopped

NON-FAST DAY
Add soba or other
wholegrain noodles.

Meatballs make hugely satisfying comfort food, and in this keto-friendly recipe they are bursting with umami and a hint of heat.

1. Preheat the oven to 200°C/Fan 180°C/Gas 6 and line a baking tray with baking parchment.

2. Combine the pork, ginger, chilli flakes, coriander and sesame oil in a bowl and mix well with your hands. Squeeze tightly to help bind the meat together.

3. Shape the mixture into 16 balls, each the size of a large cherry, and place on the prepared baking tray. Cook in the oven for 12 minutes.

4. Meanwhile, make the broth. Place the mushrooms and oil in a saucepan over a medium heat and fry for 1¼ minutes, stirring often. Stir in the miso and soy and pour in 600ml water. Bring to the boil. Reduce the heat and simmer very gently.

5. A few minutes before the pork balls are ready, add the pak choi to the broth. Simmer for 1 minute. Sprinkle in the spring onion, add the pork balls and serve immediately.

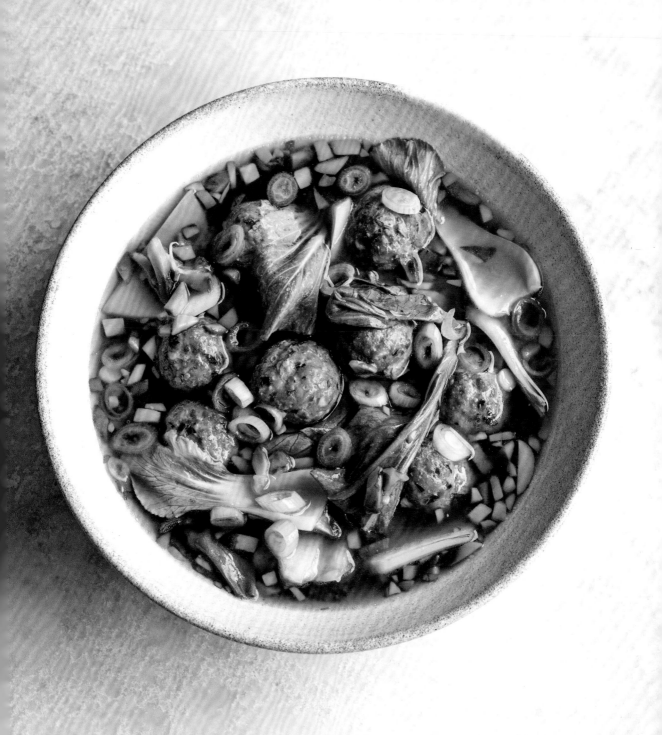

PER SERVING | **525cals** | PROTEIN **22.7g** | CARBS **15.2g**

One Pan Squeezed Sausage Casserole

SERVES	PREP	COOK
2	**10** mins	**10** mins

4 good-quality sausages
   (approx. 270g total weight)
2 tbsp olive oil
½ onion, peeled and
   thinly sliced
200g butternut squash,
   peeled and cut into 1cm dice
   (or buy ready-prepared)
½ tsp dried thyme
150g cavolo nero, central stalks
   removed and leaves sliced
1 tbsp cider vinegar
½ tsp chilli flakes (optional)

NON-FAST DAY
Increase the portion
size and/or serve with
2–3 tablespoons cooked
pearl barley or quinoa.

Oh, the joy of easy one-pan cooking!

1. Use a knife to split the skin on each sausage and remove. Cut the sausage meat into 2cm pieces.

2. Heat the oil in a large frying pan over a high heat and add the sausage pieces, onion and squash. Cook for a few minutes until slightly browned.

3. Reduce the heat to medium and stir in the thyme. Cook for 3 minutes, then add the greens, cider vinegar and chilli, if using. Cook for a final 4 minutes to soften the greens. Season with salt and black pepper to taste.

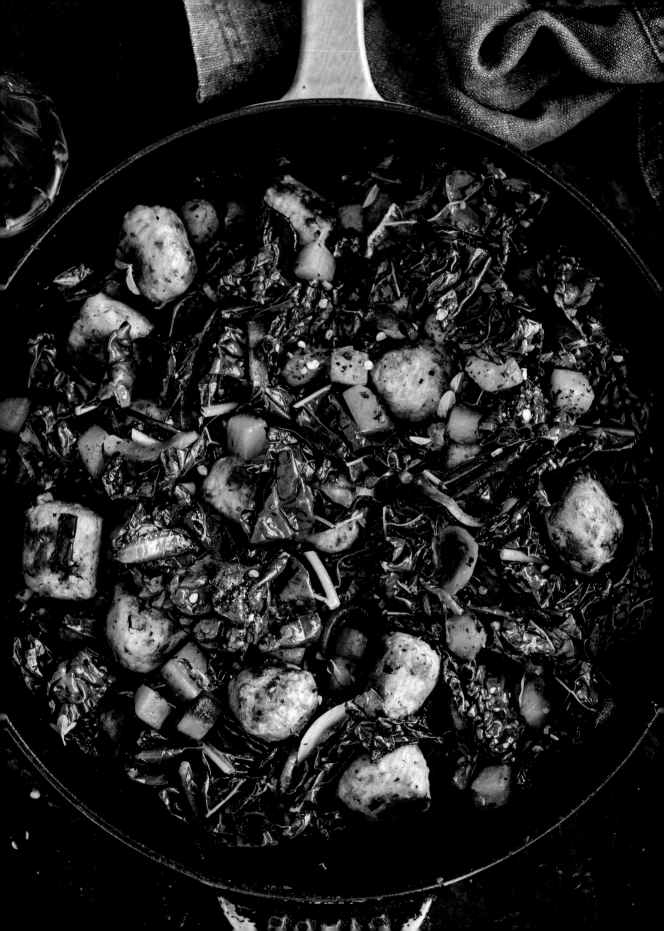

PER SERVING | **420cals** | PROTEIN **48.7g** | CARBS **12.6g**

Baked Pork with Winter Vegetables

SERVES	PREP	COOK
2	**10** mins	**30** mins

1 large leek, trimmed and
   chopped into chunks
1 large fennel bulb, trimmed
   and chopped into chunks
250g celeriac, peeled and
   chopped into chunks
4 sticks celery, chopped
   into chunks
1 tbsp olive oil
1 tsp mixed herbs
1 garlic clove, peeled
   and finely sliced
2 pork chops (approx.
   200g each), untrimmed
½ dessert apple, cored
   and thinly sliced
30g capers
100ml chicken or vegetable
   stock (made with
   ¼ stock cube)

NON-FAST DAY
Increase the portion size
and/or serve with a few
small, unpeeled baby
potatoes or Green Cauli
Mash (see page 182).

Succulent and filling, this baked pork takes on a
savoury-sweet taste when roasted alongside the
caramelised veg. Serve with half a plate of dark
greens, such as sliced cavalo nero, Swiss chard
or spring greens.

1. Preheat the oven to 200°C/Fan 180°C/Gas 6.

2. Place all the vegetables in a large bowl with the olive
oil. Season with salt and freshly ground black pepper
and add the herbs and garlic. Mix well so that everything
is lightly coated. Tip into a baking tray to fit snugly and
roast in the oven for 10 minutes.

3. Meanwhile, dry-fry the pork chops in a non-stick pan
over a medium heat for 2 minutes on each side to brown.

4. Remove the tray of vegetables from the oven and
add the apple and capers. Place the pork chops on top,
then pour in the stock. Return to the oven and bake
for a further 20 minutes, or until nicely browned.

Easy Sausage Traybake with White Beans

1 medium red onion, peeled
    and cut into 12 wedges
½ × 400g tin chopped tomatoes
1 medium red pepper, deseeded
    and cut into 3cm chunks
4 good-quality chipolata
    sausages (approx. 125g
    total weight)
1 tbsp olive oil
1 tsp hot smoked paprika
½ × 400g tin white beans
    (such as cannellini), drained
    and rinsed (approx. 120g
    drained weight)
200ml chicken or vegetable
    stock (made with
    ½ stock cube)
100g fresh spinach

NON-FAST DAY
Double the portion
and/or serve alongside
2–3 tablespoons cooked
brown rice or quinoa.

Great family food, and an ideal way to sneak in those gut-friendly beans with all that fabulous fibre. Add sliced cooked leafy greens and, if you have calories to spare, consider serving with Garlicky Mashed Turnips and Cauliflower (see page 182).

1. Preheat the oven to 200°C/Fan 180°C/Gas 6.

2. Place the onion, tomatoes, pepper and sausages on a large baking tray. Drizzle with the oil and toss lightly. Sprinkle with paprika, season with salt and lots of freshly ground black pepper and roast in the oven for 10 minutes.

3. Remove from the oven, add the beans and stock and mix well. Return to the oven and roast for 10 minutes, until the sausages are cooked through.

4. Stir the spinach into the hot sauce to wilt, and serve.

PER SERVING | **470cals** | PROTEIN **28.5g** | CARBS **26.1g**

Cheesy Fajita Beef Casserole

SERVES	PREP	COOK
4	**5–7** mins	**30** mins

1½ tbsp olive oil

1 red onion, peeled and finely chopped

2 red peppers, deseeded and finely chopped

250g minced beef

1 × 400g tin black beans, drained

2 tbsp fajita seasoning

1 × 400g tin chopped tomatoes

2 tbsp jalapeño peppers, diced

120g Cheddar, grated

4 tbsp Greek yoghurt

NON-FAST DAY
Increase the portion size and/or serve with 2–3 tablespoons cooked wholegrain rice and guacamole.

Forget starchy tacos and switch to this tasty, Mexican-inspired, fajita-flavoured casserole. You can prepare this ahead of time, leaving nothing to do other than pop the dish in the oven after a long day. Serve with fresh cooked greens.

1. Preheat the oven to 200°C/Fan 180°C/Gas 6.

2. Place a wide-based ovenproof casserole over a medium heat. Add the oil, onion and peppers and sauté for 3–4 minutes, stirring from time to time. Add the minced beef and fry for about 4 minutes, stirring to break the meat up into small pieces.

3. Stir in the black beans, fajita seasoning, tomatoes and jalapeño peppers. Simmer for 3 minutes and season well with salt and freshly ground black pepper.

4. Scatter the cheese all over and bake in the oven for 20 minutes, or until the cheese is browned and bubbling.

5. Serve with the yoghurt alongside.

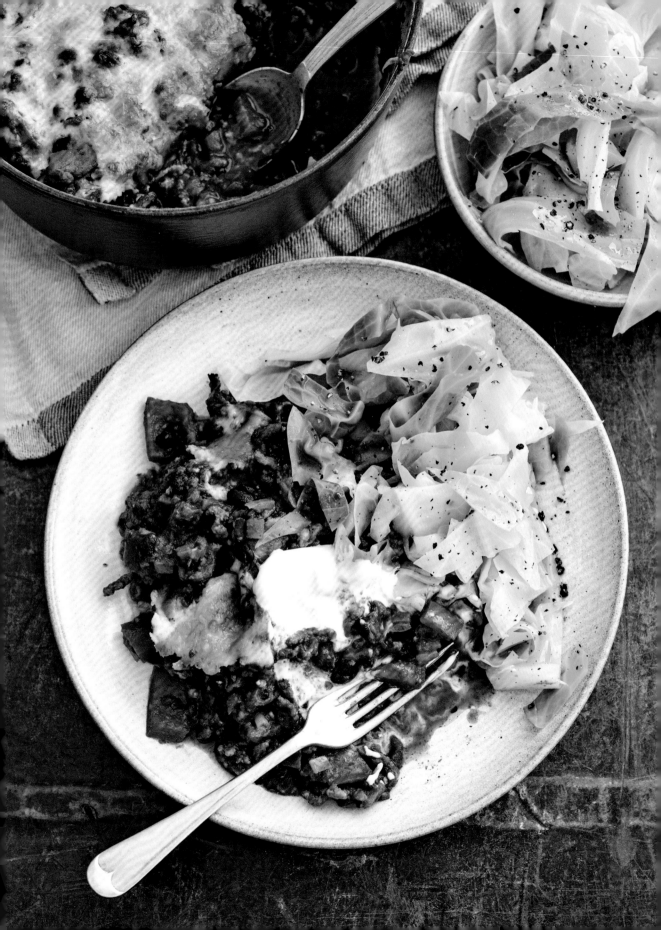

PER SERVING | **594cals** | PROTEIN **57.1g** | CARBS **5.9g**

Chargrilled Rib-eye Steak with Romesco and Broccoli

SERVES	PREP	COOK
1	**5** mins	**5–7** mins

1 rib-eye steak (approx. 227g),
   at room temperature
1 tbsp olive oil
150g tenderstem broccoli
2 tbsp Romesco Sauce
   (see below)

NON-FAST DAY
Serve with baked
celeriac chips or mash.

Spanish flavours of paprika, garlic and roasted red pepper marry beautifully with a juicy rib-eye steak.

1. Place a chargrill pan or large frying pan over a high heat.

2. Brush the steak with the olive oil and season with salt and lots of freshly ground black pepper. When the pan is smoking hot, add the steak and fry on each side for 2½ minutes for medium or 3 minutes for well done. Set aside and cover with foil to rest.

3. Meanwhile, cook the broccoli in boiling water for 2 minutes, then drain.

4. Serve the rib-eye steak with the broccoli and the Romesco Sauce alongside.

PER 1 TABLESPOON SERVING | **59cals** | PROTEIN **1.3g** | CARBS **0.7g**

Romesco Sauce

MAKES	PREP
175g	**7–10** mins

50g flaked almonds
1 roasted red pepper
   from a jar (approx. 70g)
1 garlic clove, peeled
1 tbsp tomato purée
1 tbsp cider vinegar
1 tsp smoked paprika
½ tsp cayenne pepper
3 tbsp olive oil

Served with steamed greens, this simple sauce will make a very quick and easy meal in its own right. It can also be used as a sauce for meat, fish or chicken. Or it can be drizzled onto a wrap, alongside cheese, or used as a dip for crudités. It is as delicious as it is versatile.

1. Place all of the ingredients in a small food processor with a pinch of salt and freshly ground black pepper and blitz until smooth.

2. Store in an airtight container in the fridge for up to a week. It is also suitable for freezing.

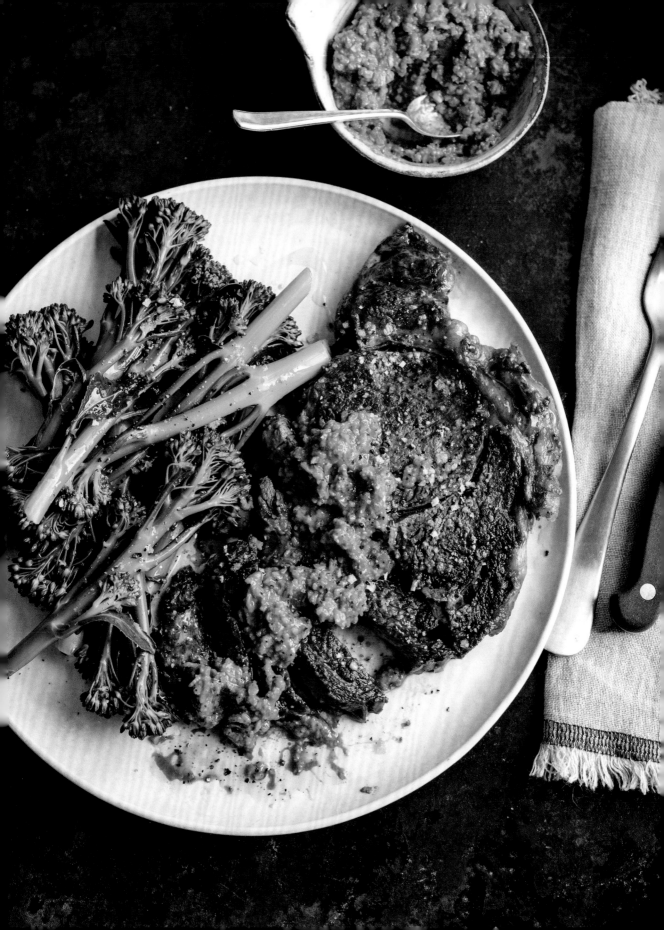

Stir-fried Beef with Broccoli

SERVES	PREP	COOK
2	**15** mins	**8** mins

400g broccoli, cut into
    small 2cm florets
3 tbsp soy sauce
Juice of 1 lime
2 garlic cloves, peeled
    and finely chopped
15g fresh root ginger,
    peeled and grated
1 small red chilli, seeds
    removed if you want less
    spice and finely chopped
1 tbsp rapeseed (ideally
    cold-pressed) or olive oil
1 rump steak, thinly sliced
    (approx. 250g)

COOK'S TIP

For a vegan version, replace
the beef with 230g edamame
beans (370cals, 27g protein
and 24g carbs per serving).

NON-FAST DAY

Increase the portion
size and/or serve with
2–3 tablespoons cooked
wholegrain rice or soba
or brown noodles.

We love last-minute stir-fries. Beef and broccoli,
flavoured with garlic, ginger and a bit of chilli, is
a winning combination. This recipe is high in fibre
and surprisingly keto-friendly if you serve it with
extra cooked greens and cauli-rice (see page 68).

1. Place the broccoli in a medium bowl and cover with
boiling water. Cover the bowl and leave for 5 minutes.

2. Meanwhile, mix the soy sauce, lime juice, garlic,
ginger and chilli together in a bowl.

3. Place the oil in a wok or heavy-based frying pan over
a high heat. When it is smoking hot, add the steak and
stir-fry for 1½ minutes. Remove the steak from the
pan and set aside.

4. Drain the broccoli and add it to the wok with a splash
of water. Stir-fry for 2–3 minutes, then pour in the sauce
and simmer for 1 minute.

5. Remove the pan from the heat and stir in the
cooked steak.

Roasted Pork Fillet with Mediterranean Veg

SERVES **4**

PREP **15** mins

COOK **30** mins

1 tsp paprika

2 tbsp olive oil

1 × 350g pork loin

1 courgette, halved lengthwise and sliced into 1cm half moons

2 medium red peppers, deseeded and sliced into 2cm wedges

1 aubergine, cut into 2cm pieces

2 tbsp balsamic vinegar

2 level tbsp sun-dried tomato pesto

½–1 tsp Dijon mustard

COOK'S TIP

A handful of rocket dressed with a little oil and lemon juice would make a nice addition.

NON-FAST DAY

Double the portion size and drizzle with olive oil to serve. You could also serve 2–3 tablespoons cooked wholegrains, such as rice, bulgur wheat or quinoa, alongside, or with slices of baked butternut squash.

Pork loin is readily available and a very affordable cut of meat, and here, teamed with delicious Mediterranean flavours, makes a quick and easy mid-week meal, as well as a great Sunday roast. Serve on a generous bed of rocket, spinach and/or watercress, or alongside a colourful leafy salad.

1. Preheat the oven to 220°C/Fan 200°C/Gas 8 and line a large baking tray with baking parchment.

2. Mix the paprika with ½ tablespoon of the olive oil and use to coat the pork loin. Season well with salt and freshly ground black pepper.

3. Place the courgette, peppers and aubergine on one side of the prepared tray. Drizzle with 1 tablespoon of the oil and season.

4. Place a frying pan over a very high heat with the remaining oil. When the oil is smoking, sear the pork on all sides for 2–3 minutes, until it is nicely browned. Transfer to the tray with the vegetables and roast in the oven for 30 minutes. Remove the pork and set aside to rest for about 5 minutes before slicing.

5. Meanwhile, mix the balsamic vinegar, sun-dried tomato pesto and mustard together in a bowl. Serve the pork and roasted vegetables with the balsamic and sun-dried tomato sauce drizzled on top.

PER SERVING | **482cals** | PROTEIN **39.6g** | CARBS **19.3g**

Navarin of Lamb with Mangetout

SERVES	PREP	COOK
2	**10** mins	**105** mins

2 tbsp olive oil
350g diced lamb shoulder
1 medium red onion,
   peeled and sliced
2 garlic cloves, peeled
   and finely chopped
6 sprigs of thyme, leaves
   picked (or 1 tsp dried)
1 tbsp tomato purée
1 beef stock cube
250g butternut squash,
   peeled and sliced
100g mangetout

NON-FAST DAY
Increase the portion size and
serve with 2–3 tablespoons
wholegrains, such as pearl
barley or bulgur wheat.

Traditionally a navarin of lamb is made using root vegetables. Here, lighter, less starchy spring vegetables are used instead – you could also use green beans, runner beans or sliced savoy cabbage. A deeply satisfying stew which is easy to put together. Serve with Green Cauli Mash (see page 182).

1. Preheat the oven to 180°C/Fan 160°C/Gas 4.

2. Place ½ tablespoon of the oil in a heavy-based medium ovenproof saucepan with a lid over a high heat. When hot, place a single layer of diced lamb in the pan (it is important not to overcrowd the pan, or the meat will stew.) Brown for a couple of minutes, then turn. Remove the meat from the pan and repeat with the remaining lamb and another ½ tablespoon of the oil. Remove the second batch and set aside.

3. Add the remaining oil to the pan and stir in the onion. Add a splash of water, cover with a lid and sweat for 3 minutes. Add the garlic and thyme and cook uncovered for 30 seconds. Stir in the tomato purée, crumble in the stock cube and pour in 400ml water. Return the lamb to the pan, bring to a simmer, cover with the lid and transfer to the oven for 1½ hours.

4. Halfway through the cooking time, add the butternut squash and season with salt and freshly ground black pepper.

5. Remove from the oven and add the mangetout – the heat from the stew will be enough to cook them.

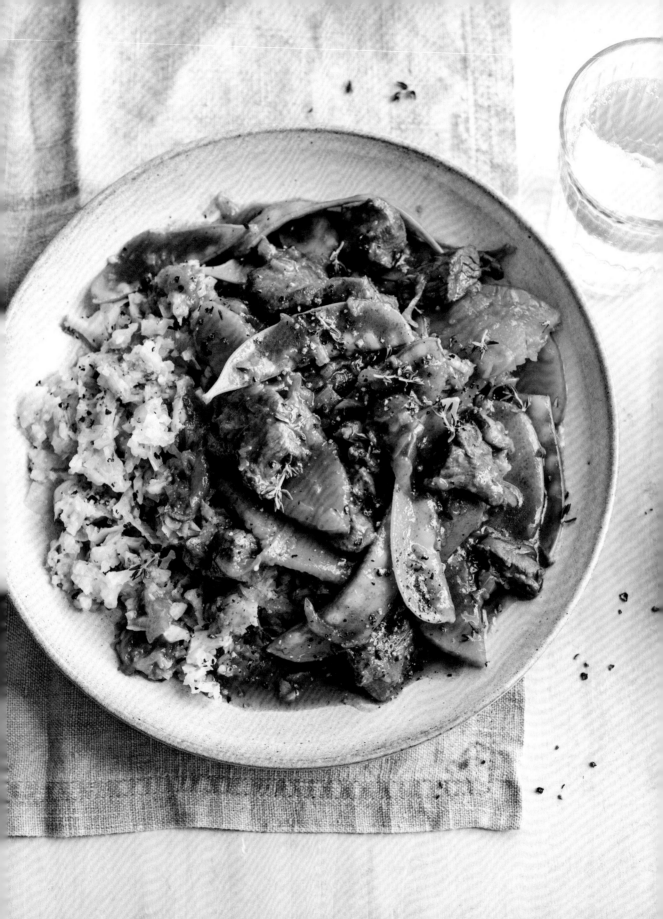

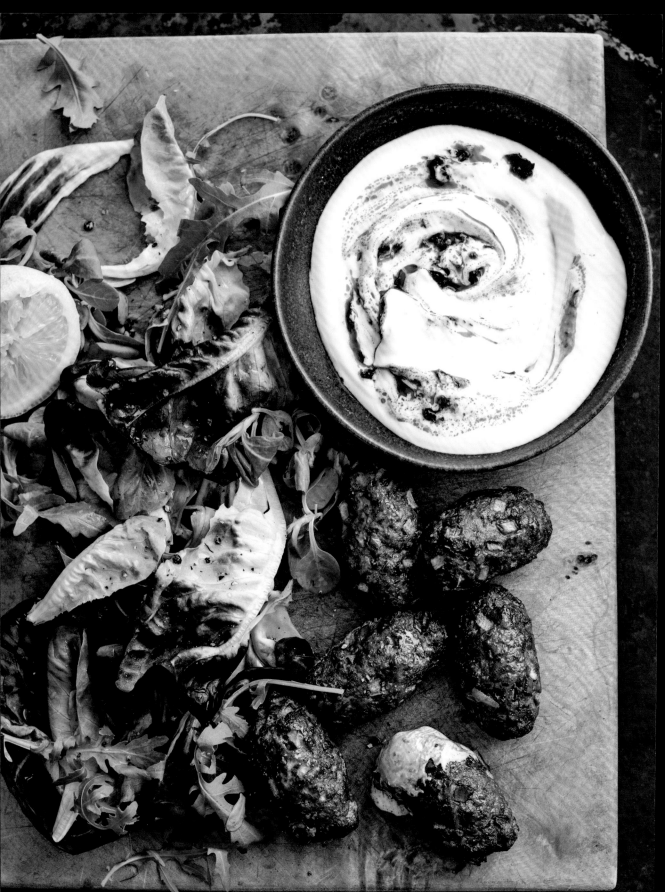

Easy Lamb Koftas with Green Salad and Harissa Yoghurt

SERVES | **PREP** | **COOK**
2 | **10–15** mins | **15** mins

250g minced lamb
½ red onion, peeled
　and finely chopped
1 garlic clove, peeled
　and finely chopped
½ tsp dried oregano
½ tsp ground cumin
½ tsp ground cinnamon
　(optional)
5g fresh flat-leaf parsley,
　finely chopped
4 tbsp full-fat Greek yoghurt
1 tbsp harissa paste
150g mixed salad leaves
1 tsp olive oil
1 tsp fresh lemon juice

COOK'S TIP
These can be made
a day ahead or frozen
for a later date.

NON-FAST DAY
Serve with 2–3 tablespoons
cooked quinoa, bulgur wheat
or a wholegrain pitta.

These mildly spiced, sausage-shaped koftas deliver delicious Middle Eastern flavours with the minimum of effort. They also make a great on-the-go lunch.

1. Preheat the oven to 200°C/Fan 180°C/Gas 6 and line a baking tray with baking parchment.

2. Place the lamb, red onion, garlic, oregano, cumin, cinnamon, if using, and parsley in a bowl with a generous pinch of salt and freshly ground black pepper. Use your hands to mix everything together.

3. Divide the lamb mixture into six pieces and shape each one into a 7.5cm sausage shape. Place on the prepared baking tray and cook in the oven for 15 minutes.

4. Meanwhile, mix the yoghurt and harissa together in a small bowl with a pinch of salt.

5. Toss the leaves in the olive oil and lemon juice, season and serve with the koftas and the harissa yoghurt alongside.

PER SERVING | **415cals** | PROTEIN **38.9g** | CARBS **6.8g**

Tandoori Lamb Cutlets with Garlic and Ginger Spinach

SERVES **2** | PREP **10** mins | COOK **12** mins

2 tbsp full-fat Greek yoghurt

1 tbsp tandoori powder

4 lamb chops
    (approx. 75g each)

1 tbsp olive oil

1 garlic clove, peeled
    and roughly chopped

10g fresh root ginger,
    peeled and grated

350g fresh spinach

15g cashew nuts,
    roughly chopped

NON-FAST DAY
Increase the portion size and serve with 2–3 tablespoons of cooked wholegrains, such as brown rice.

Thanks to tandoori seasoning, lamb chops just got more interesting. This is a simple dish packed with flavour.

1. Preheat the grill to its highest setting and line a baking tray with baking parchment.

2. Mix the yoghurt with the tandoori powder in a large bowl and season with salt and freshly ground black pepper. Add the lamb chops and toss to coat. Place on the prepared baking tray and cook under the grill for 6 minutes on each side. Set aside to rest for a couple of minutes.

3. Meanwhile, place the olive oil in a large frying pan over a medium heat. Add the garlic and ginger and sauté for 1 minute. Add the spinach and stir to wilt the leaves – this will take 1–2 minutes. Season and keep warm.

4. Divide the spinach between two warm plates, scatter the cashew nuts all over and place the lamb chops on top to serve.

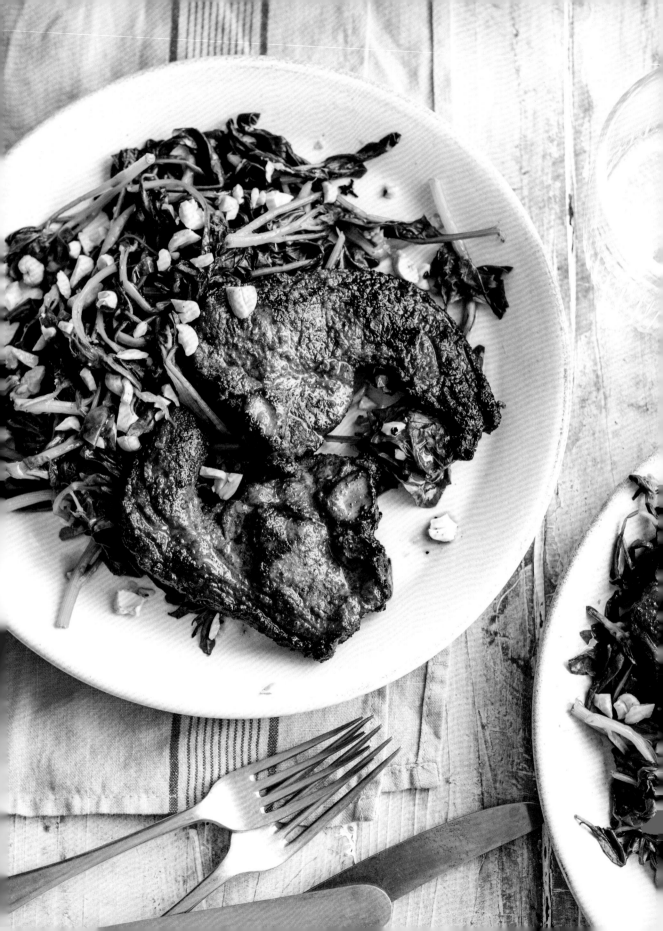

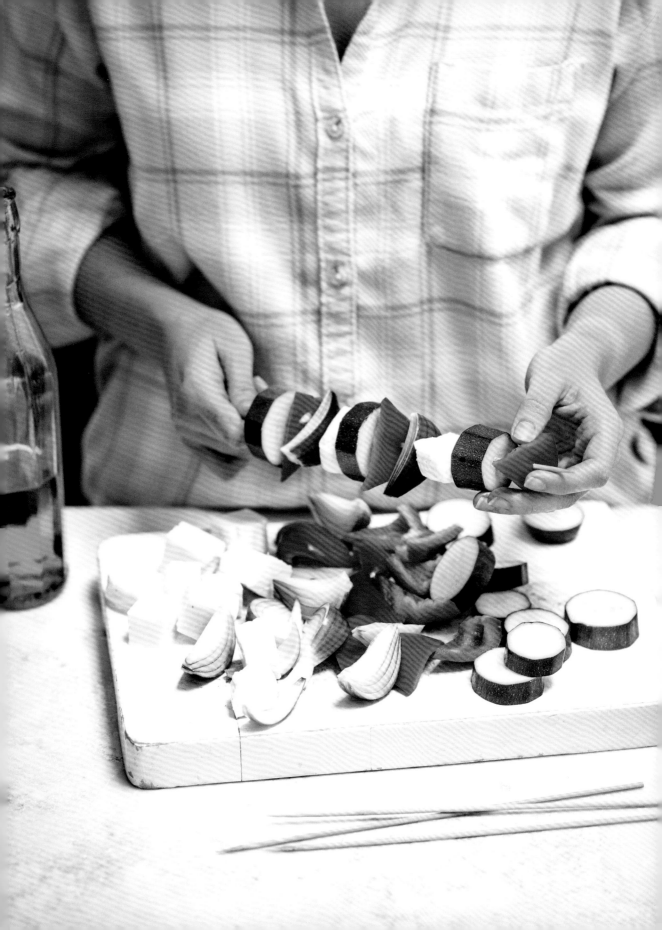

Meat-free

Following a keto diet as a vegetarian has
never been so easy... You will find lots
of one-pan meals here. And remember,
for extra protein you can make use of our
no-count protein top-ups (see page 240).
The more variety of veg you eat the better,
ideally aiming for 30 different types over
the course of a week. This can include herbs.

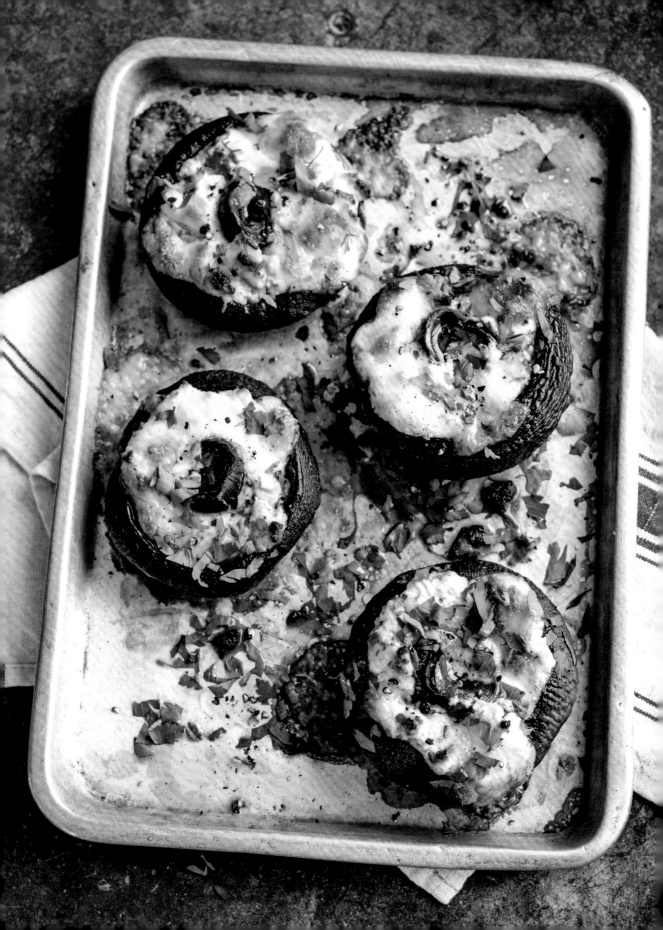

Easy Garlicky Mushrooms

SERVES
2

PREP
15
mins

COOK
15
mins

4 large mushrooms
(approx. 65g each)
75g Garlic and Herb Boursin
½ ball mozzarella (approx.
75g), torn into small pieces
Small handful flat-leaf parsley,
roughly chopped

NON-FAST DAY
Serve the mushrooms
on seeded sourdough or
toasted wholegrain bread.

Who can resist baked garlicky mushrooms? These are like mini low-carb pizzas, but without the starchy base and all the better for it! Scatter with parsley, if you have it, and serve with a large colourful salad.

1. Preheat the oven to 190°C/Fan 170°C/Gas 5 and line a baking tray with baking parchment.

2. Place the mushrooms on the tray and divide the Boursin between them. Top with the mozzarella, season with plenty of freshly ground black pepper and a little salt to taste. Bake in the oven for 15 minutes, until the cheese has melted and is golden brown in places.

3. Scatter with the parsley to serve.

Warm Orange and Walnut Salad with Halloumi

SERVES	PREP	COOK
2	**15** mins	**5** mins

30g walnuts or pecans
115g halloumi, diced
1 tbsp olive oil
40g rocket
2 heads of red chicory,
   leaves removed and
   each sliced into 3
1 medium orange, skin and
   pith removed, thinly sliced

For the Dijon dressing:
1 tbsp extra-virgin olive oil
1 tbsp cider vinegar
1 tsp wholegrain or smooth
   Dijon mustard

COOK'S TIP
Red blush oranges
in season add a little
magic to this recipe!

NON-FAST DAY
Serve a double portion
with 2–3 tablespoons
cooked wholegrains.

Fruit – particularly lower sugar varieties such as hard pears, apples, oranges and berries – is an important part of our diet, but is best eaten with or straight after a meal, as this dramatically reduces the sugar spike. Here the orange not only creates a superb sweet and tangy flavour in contrast to the bitter salad leaves, but also delivers much-needed nutrients and fibre.

1. Start by making the dressing. Whisk all the ingredients together until emulsified. Season with salt and freshly ground black pepper.

2. Toast the walnuts or pecans in a dry frying pan over a medium heat for 1–2 minutes. Set aside.

3. Use the same pan to fry the halloumi in the oil over a medium heat for 2–3 minutes, until just starting to turn golden brown.

4. Toss the rocket and chicory in the dressing and divide between two plates. Top with the halloumi, orange slices and toasted nuts to serve.

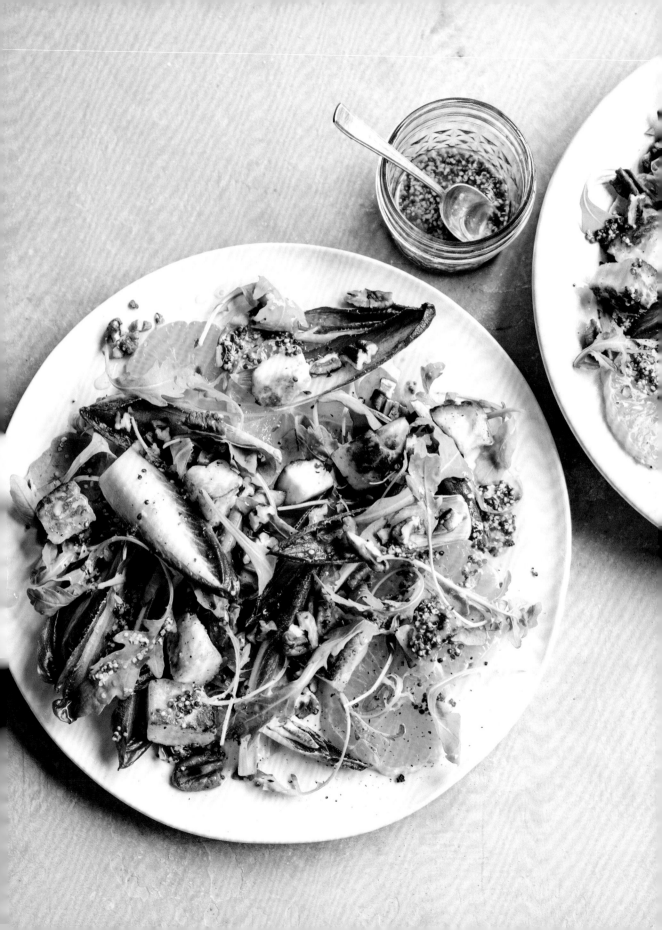

Roasted Mediterranean Veg with Tapenade and Mozzarella

SERVES 2 | **PREP** 10 mins | **COOK** 30 mins

1 small aubergine,
    cut into 2cm chunks
1 small bulb of fennel,
    quartered and cut into
    2cm chunks
1 small red pepper,
    cut into 2cm chunks
½ medium red onion, peeled
    and sliced into wedges
2 tbsp olive oil
1 heaped tbsp black olive
    tapenade (approx. 20g)
1 tsp fresh lemon juice
125g ball of mozzarella,
    roughly torn
25g flaked almonds
10g basil, leaves picked
    (optional)

NON-FAST DAY
Double the portion size,
add an extra glug of olive
oil and choose some protein
top-ups (see page 240).

Tapenade, a spread made from puréed olives, has a gorgeous savoury, tangy flavour and makes this tray of Mediterranean vegetables utterly delicious.

1. Preheat the oven to 220°C/Fan 200°C/Gas 8.

2. Place the vegetables in a medium roasting dish and toss with 1 tablespoon of the olive oil. Season well with salt and freshly ground black pepper and roast in the oven for 25 minutes.

3. Mix the remaining olive oil with the tapenade and lemon juice in a small bowl until smooth.

4. Carefully remove the dish from the oven and pour the dressing all over. Toss to coat. Scatter the mozzarella all over and return to the oven for 5 minutes, or until the cheese has melted.

5. Sprinkle with the almonds and fresh basil, if using, to serve.

Green Vegetable Gratin

SERVES | PREP | COOK
4 | **10** mins | **20** mins

1 tsp butter, for greasing
2 large leeks, trimmed
   and sliced
100g cavolo nero,
   roughly chopped
125ml hot vegetable stock
   (made with ¼ stock cube)
125ml crème fraîche
2 tsp Dijon mustard
50g Parmesan, grated
100g hazelnuts,
   roughly chopped
30g Cheddar, grated

NON-FAST DAY
Serve with a slice of
toasted seeded sourdough
or wholemeal seeded bread,
and add a protein top-up
or two (see page 240).

Luscious creamy baked veg coated in a cheesy sauce,
topped with crunchy toasted hazelnuts. A meal on its
own but you could turbo-charge your protein intake
by adding a protein top-up too (see page 240).

1. Preheat the oven to 200°C/Fan 180°C/Gas 6 and butter
a gratin or pie dish.

2. Steam or blanch the leeks and cavolo nero for a couple
of minutes to soften, then drain.

3. Place the vegetables and the hot stock in the prepared
gratin or pie dish. Season with a pinch of salt and freshly
ground black pepper.

4. Combine the crème fraiche, mustard and Parmesan in
a small bowl. Stir the sauce into the veg so everything is
lightly coated. Scatter the nuts and Cheddar over the top
and bake in the oven for 15 minutes, or until beginning
to colour and the cheese is melting.

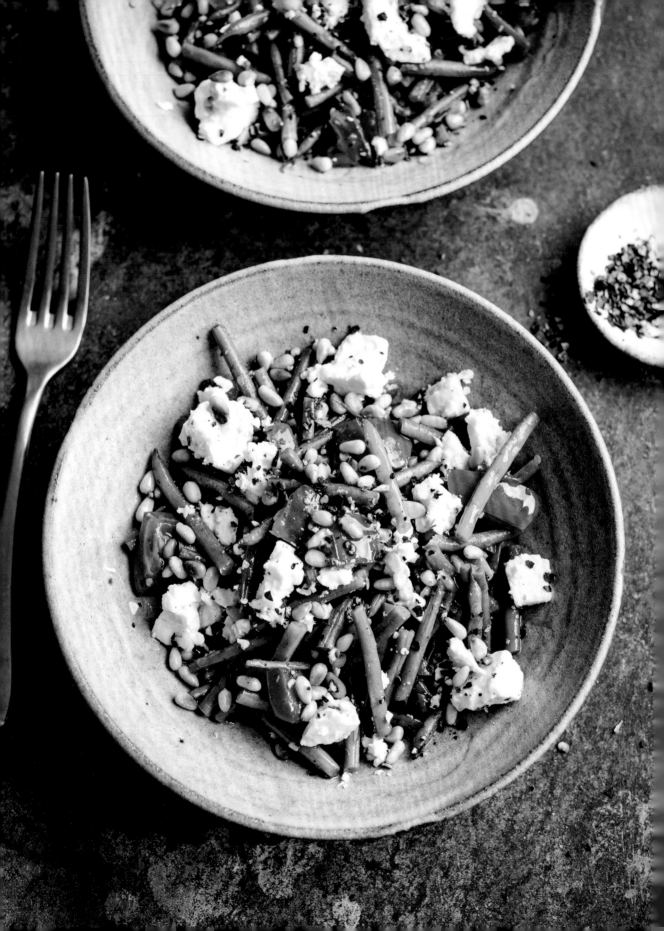

French Bean Bowl with Feta and Pine Nuts

SERVES
2

PREP
10 mins

COOK
10 mins

2 tbsp pine nuts
  (or other seeds)
180g French beans,
  topped, tailed and
  cut into 2cm pieces
1 tbsp olive oil
2 medium tomatoes,
  cut into 2cm pieces
1 garlic clove, peeled
  and finely chopped
100g feta cheese,
  roughly crumbled
Pinch of chilli flakes
  (optional)

NON-FAST DAY
Increase the portion size.

Although not a great gardener, I do like growing beans. Beans are a good source of soluble and insoluble fibre, and their juicy crunch contrasts beautifully here with the salty, creamy feta. I try to keep a pack of feta in the fridge – it's great for adding a flavourful protein boost to salads and oven bakes. This dish would work well in a lunchbox.

1. Place the pine nuts in a dry frying pan over a medium heat and toast for 1–2 minutes, or until turning golden. Remove from the pan and set aside.

2. Return the pan to the heat, add the beans and oil and fry for a couple of minutes, stirring occasionally. Stir in the tomatoes and cook for 4 minutes. Add the garlic and cook for 1 minute more. Remove from the heat and scatter the feta and pine nuts all over.

3. Allow to rest for a minute or so, to let the feta soften, then divide between two bowls and season with plenty of freshly ground black pepper and a pinch of chilli flakes, if using.

PER SERVING | **457cals** | PROTEIN **17.9g** | CARBS **14g**

Roasted Veg with Feta, Almonds and Red Pepper Sauce

SERVES | PREP | COOK
2 | **10–15** mins | **30** mins

1 medium aubergine,
   cut into 2cm dice
½ small cauliflower,
   florets, leaves and stalks
   all roughly chopped
1 tsp fennel seeds (optional)
1½ tbsp olive oil
100g feta cheese, crumbled
2 tbsp flaked almonds
   (approx. 35g)

*For the roasted red pepper
   and balsamic sauce:*
1 roasted red pepper
   from a jar (approx. 70g)
1 tbsp balsamic vinegar
1 tbsp olive oil
¼ tsp chilli flakes

NON-FAST DAY
Increase the portion size
and serve with a wholegrain
pitta, or 2–3 tablespoons
cooked wholegrains.

A traybake of roasted veg is so easy and satisfying. Roasted cauli turns sweet and juicy, while aubergine becomes slightly scorched with creamy flesh. With a drizzle of roasted pepper sauce and a scattering of toasted almonds, you have a healthy feast!

1. Preheat the oven to 220°C/Fan 200°C/Gas 8.

2. Place the aubergine and cauliflower in a medium baking dish, scatter the fennel seeds all over, if using, and toss in the olive oil to coat. Season with salt and freshly ground black pepper and roast in the oven for 25 minutes, stirring halfway through.

3. Meanwhile, place the sauce ingredients in a bowl or jug and blitz with a stick blender until the pepper is broken down but still a little chunky.

4. Remove the veg from the oven and scatter the feta cheese over the top. Drizzle over the sauce and sprinkle with the almonds. Return to the oven for a final 5 minutes. Serve immediately.

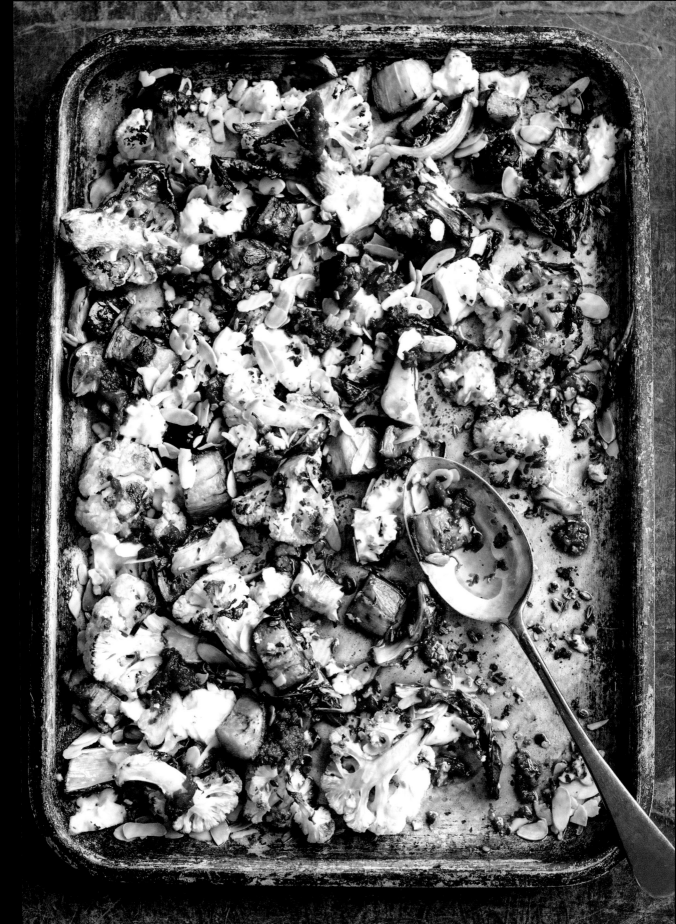

PER SERVING | **204cals** | PROTEIN **4.4g** | CARBS **1.6g**

Spring Green Frittata with Goat's Cheese

SERVES	PREP	COOK
4	**10** mins	**5–6** mins

2 spring onions, trimmed
    and roughly chopped
50g asparagus, woody
    ends removed, spears
    roughly chopped
60g green beans, trimmed
    and roughly chopped
1 tbsp olive oil
16g Garlic and Herb Boursin
50g spinach or rocket (or a mix
    of both), roughly chopped
6 medium free-range eggs,
    beaten
50g soft goat's cheese

COOK'S TIP

Boursin can be bought in
small individually wrapped
cubes, each weighing 16g,
which are useful to keep
in the fridge.

NON-FAST DAY

Serve a double portion
with steamed veg or salad,
and a few small unpeeled
boiled potatoes with a
dollop of butter or olive oil.

This bright and colourful frittata makes a delicious main meal and can double up as a portable lunch, as it tastes great cold, too. Boursin adds a delicious depth of flavour as well as adding protein. Serve with a generous green salad.

1. Preheat the grill to high.

2. Place all the chopped veg and olive oil in a medium non-stick frying pan and sauté over a medium heat for 2–3 minutes. Add the Boursin and the leaves and stir for about 30 seconds, until wilted. Season with a pinch of salt and freshly ground black pepper.

3. Pour in the eggs, season and cook for 3 minutes.

4. Crumble the goat's cheese all over, then place under the grill for 2–3 minutes, or until the eggs have set and browned slightly. Allow to cool a little before serving.

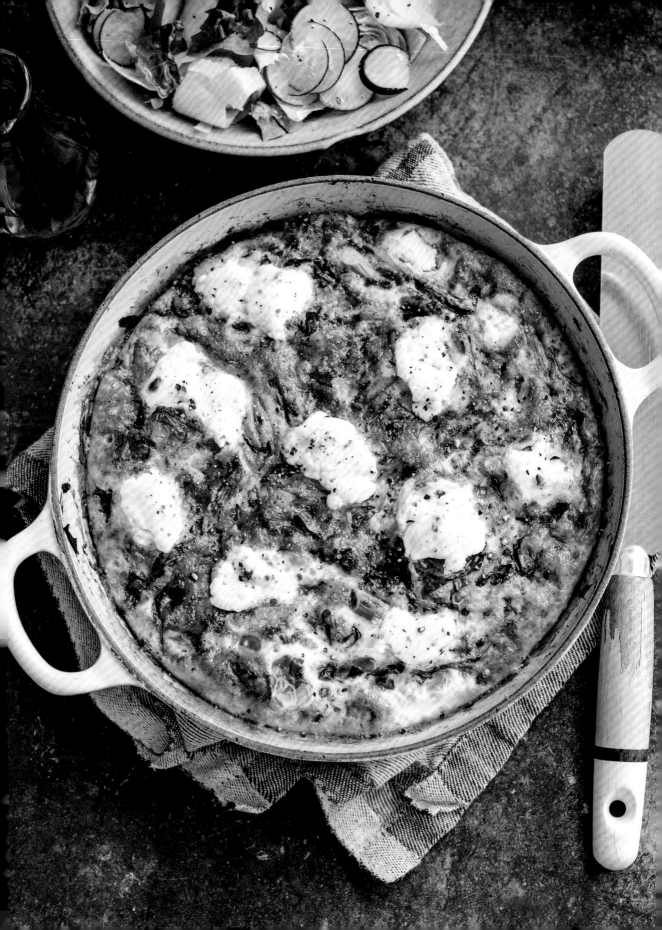

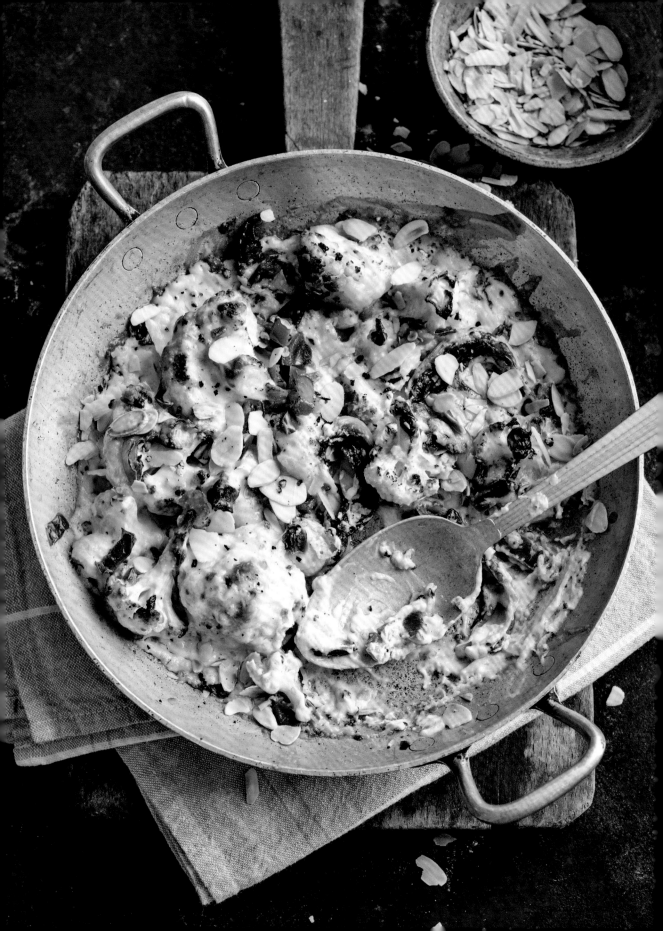

Cauli Cheese with Jalapeño Peppers

SERVES	PREP	COOK
2	**10** mins	**25** mins

½ medium cauliflower
1 tbsp olive oil
70g full-fat cream cheese
1 tbsp Dijon mustard
1½ tbsp milk
60g Cheddar, grated
30g jalapeños, roughly chopped
2 tbsp toasted flaked almonds
   (approx. 35g)

COOK'S TIP
For non-vegetarians, this dish is lovely served with cured hams, diced bacon or chorizo (see protein top-ups on page 240).

NON-FAST DAY
Serve a larger portion and add extra cheese.

Forget stodgy bechamel sauce. This quick and fuss-free version of cauliflower cheese is juicy and creamy, and nicely balanced by a mild spicy kick from the jalapeño peppers. A fabulous, easy mid-week meal. Serve with steamed greens or a colourful leafy salad if you like.

1. Preheat the oven to 200°C/Fan 180°C/Gas 6.

2. Chop the cauliflower stalks and florets into small chunks. Place in a medium baking dish and toss with the olive oil. Season with salt and freshly ground black pepper and roast in the oven for 15 minutes.

3. Meanwhile, in a small bowl, mix together the cream cheese, mustard, milk and half of the Cheddar. Remove the dish from the oven and stir in the cream cheese mixture. Scatter the jalapeños all over, along with the remaining grated cheese. Season with a little more salt and lots of freshly ground black pepper and return to the oven for a further 10–15 minutes, until golden and bubbling.

4. Garnish with the flaked almonds to serve.

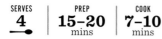

Halloumi Skewers with Coleslaw

SERVES
4

PREP
15–20 mins

COOK
7–10 mins

1 × 225g pack halloumi,
   cut into 12
1 small courgette, cut into 12
1 small red pepper, deseeded
   and cut into 12
½ red onion, peeled and
   cut into 12
1½ tbsp olive oil
1 batch Simple Coleslaw
   (see page 193)

NON-FAST DAY
Double the portion size and
serve with 2–3 tablespoons
cooked wholegrains, such
as quinoa, bulgur wheat
or brown rice.

Halloumi, unlike most other cheeses, remains
firm when fried or griddled and browns beautifully,
making it ideal to add flavour and protein to kebabs.
This gorgeous summery dish will also work really
well on a barbeque.

1. Soak 4 wooden skewers in cold water for 10 minutes.

2. Divide the ingredients between the skewers and drizzle
with the olive oil. Season with a small pinch of salt and
freshly ground black pepper.

3. Place a griddle pan over a high heat and, when hot,
add the skewers and cook on each side until the veggies
are slightly charred and the halloumi is soft.

4. Serve with the coleslaw.

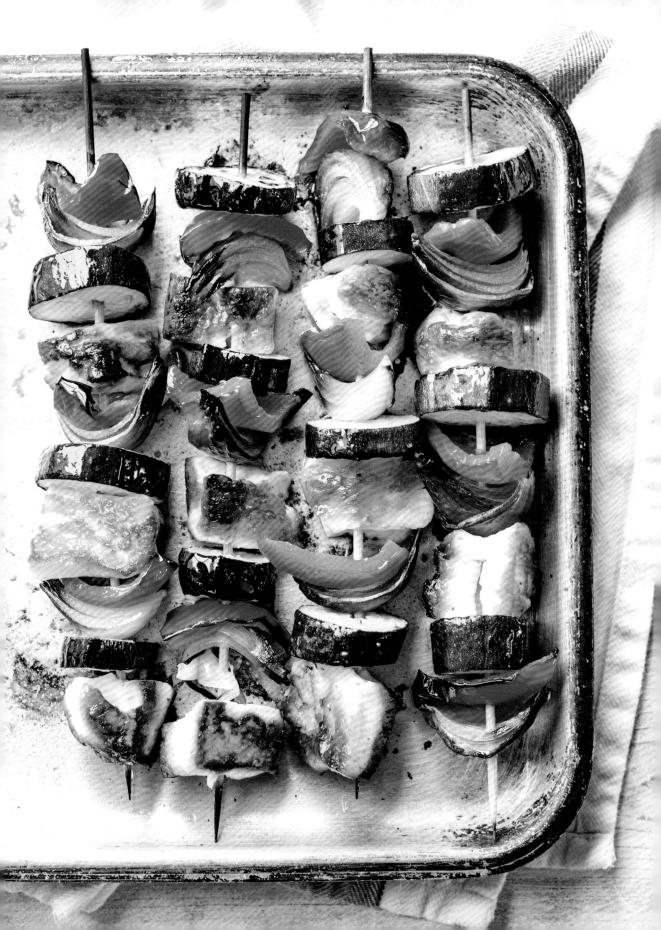

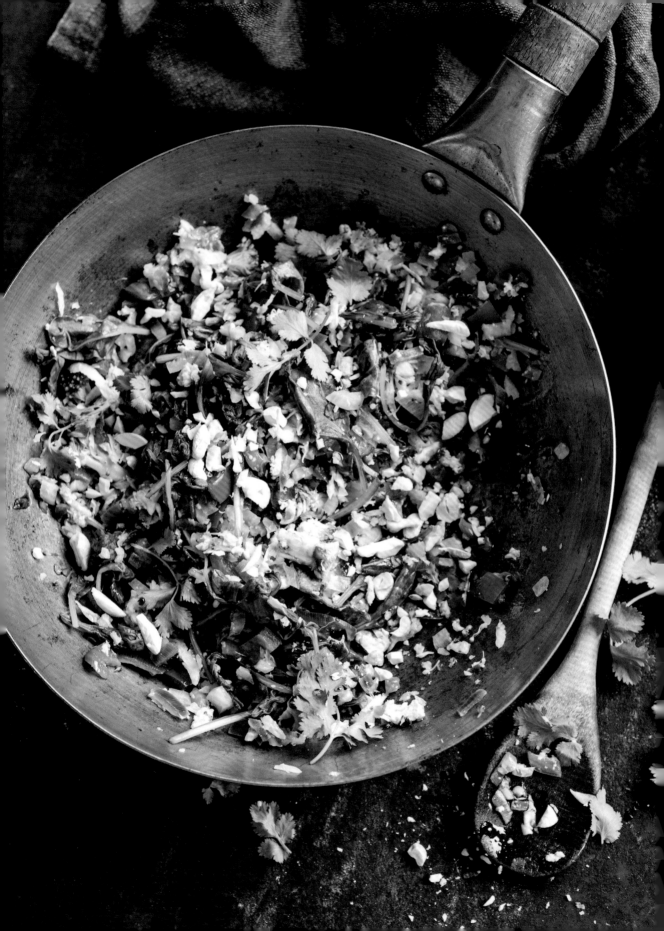

Egg-fried Cauli and Broccoli Rice

SERVES
2

PREP
10–12
mins

COOK
10
mins

1 tbsp olive oil
1 red onion, peeled
   and finely chopped
1 small red pepper,
   deseeded and diced
1 garlic clove, peeled
   and roughly chopped
1 small red chilli, finely sliced
   (or ½–1 tsp chilli flakes)
150g cauli-rice (see page 68)
   or ¼ cauliflower,
   coarsely grated
100g broccoli, coarsely grated
50g fresh spinach
2 medium free-range eggs
1½ tbsp soy sauce
10g fresh coriander,
   roughly chopped
10g cashew nuts,
   roughly chopped

NON-FAST DAY
Enjoy a larger portion
and add some protein
top-ups (see page 240).

This colourful plant-based version of egg-fried rice
is a great way to introduce a variety of vegetables
into a meal and to use up odds and ends from the
fridge. Ideally, we should all be eating at least
30 different vegetables a week.

1. Place the oil in a wok or large frying pan over a high
heat and, when hot, add the onion and pepper. Stir-fry
for 2 minutes, then add the garlic and chilli and fry for
30 seconds.

2. Stir in the cauli and broccoli and stir-fry for 3–4 minutes,
until hot and just starting to soften. Add the spinach and
stir to wilt.

3. Push everything to one side of the pan and crack in the
eggs. Stir until starting to scramble, then mix everything
together with the soy sauce. Cook for 1 minute. Finally
add the coriander and garnish with cashews to serve.

Teriyaki Tofu Stir-fry

SERVES	PREP	COOK
2	**5** mins	**10** mins

1 tbsp olive or rapeseed oil
1 small onion, peeled and diced
1 small red pepper, deseeded
    and sliced
10g fresh root ginger,
    peeled and roughly grated
200g teriyaki firm tofu,
    cut into 2cm dice
½ tsp chilli flakes (optional)
1 tsp sesame oil
200g cauli-rice (see page 68)
1 tbsp soy sauce
20g cashew nuts,
    roughly chopped
10g fresh coriander,
    roughly chopped,
    to garnish (optional)

COOK'S TIP
Packs of cauli-rice
are available in most
supermarkets.

NON-FAST DAY
Swap the cauli-rice
for 2–3 tablespoons
cooked brown rice or
wholegrain noodles.

I'm enjoying getting to know tofu as a meat alternative, and trying different flavours, and have come across a gem in this firm teriyaki variety. It has great texture and an authentic and mildly spiced flavour. If you can't find teriyaki flavour, try smoked tofu, available in most supermarkets.

1. Place the oil in a large frying pan or wok until hot, add the onion and red pepper and stir-fry for 4–5 minutes.

2. Reduce the heat to medium and add the ginger, tofu, chilli flakes, if using, and sesame oil and cook for 1 minute.

3. Stir in the cauli-rice and stir-fry for 3–4 minutes.

4. Add the soy sauce and garnish with cashew nuts and fresh coriander, if using, to serve.

Glazed Ginger and Garlic Tofu with Spinach

SERVES	PREP	COOK
2	**10** mins	**5** mins

150g frozen spinach
100g firm tofu, cut into
   2 slices about 1cm thick
1 medium free-range
   egg, whisked
1½ tbsp olive oil
2 garlic cloves, peeled
   and finely chopped
10g fresh root ginger,
   peeled and finely chopped
½ tsp chilli flakes
1 tbsp soy sauce
Juice of ½ lime
20g cashew nuts,
   roughly chopped

NON-FAST DAY
Enjoy a larger portion and serve with 2–3 tablespoons brown rice or quinoa.

This flavoursome glazed tofu would work well with any steamed greens. It will also help you get your protein fix for the day.

1. Place the spinach in a bowl and defrost in the microwave for a couple of minutes. Squeeze out excess water, season with salt and freshly ground black pepper and keep warm.

2. Place the tofu between two pieces of kitchen paper and squeeze out as much excess liquid as possible. Dip the tofu in the egg to coat.

3. Place ½ tablespoon of the olive oil in a non-stick frying pan over a high heat. Add the tofu and fry on each side for 1–2 minutes, until golden brown. Move to one side of the pan and pour in the remaining oil. Add the garlic, ginger and chilli flakes and fry for about 30 seconds, stirring all the time.

4. Add the soy sauce, mix well and toss the tofu in the sauce.

5. Squeeze the lime juice all over and place the glazed tofu and sauce on top of the warm spinach. Sprinkle with the cashew nuts to serve.

PER SERVING | **286cals** | PROTEIN **14.8g** | CARBS **19.2g**

Spiced Baked Beans with Cavolo Nero and Egg

SERVES	PREP	COOK
4	**10** mins	**15** mins

1 medium onion, peeled
    and finely diced
3 tbsp olive oil
1 large or 2 small garlic cloves,
    peeled and roughly chopped
2 tsp smoked paprika
½ tsp chilli flakes (optional)
1 × 400g tin white beans
    (such as cannelloni), drained
    and rinsed (approx. 235g
    drained weight)
1 × 400g tin chopped tomatoes
1 veg stock cube
1 tbsp balsamic vinegar
1 tsp dried oregano
200g cavolo nero, stalks
    removed and leaves
    roughly chopped
4 medium free-range eggs

NON-FAST DAY
Increase the portion
size, add an extra egg
and serve it on a slice of
toasted seeded sourdough
or wholemeal bread.

Baked bean comfort food with an egg cracked on top. With its smoky flavours, you could almost be back at the ranch. The beans are best made in advance, as their flavour develops over time. Have a batch ready in the fridge for a quick supper, lunch or breakfast.

1. Place the onion and 2 tablespoons of the olive oil in a medium saucepan over a medium heat. Sauté for about 3 minutes, until softened. Add the garlic and fry for 1 minute. Stir in the paprika and chilli flakes, if using, followed by the beans and chopped tomatoes. Sprinkle in the stock cube and stir in the balsamic vinegar and dried oregano. Bring to the boil, then reduce the heat and simmer gently for 5 minutes. Season with salt and freshly ground black pepper to taste.

2. Meanwhile, place the cavolo nero and the remaining oil in a non-stick pan and sauté for a few minutes, until softened. Divide between two plates and keep warm.

3. Crack the eggs into the pan and cook to your liking.

4. Serve a generous spoonful of beans on the cavolo nero and top with a fried egg.

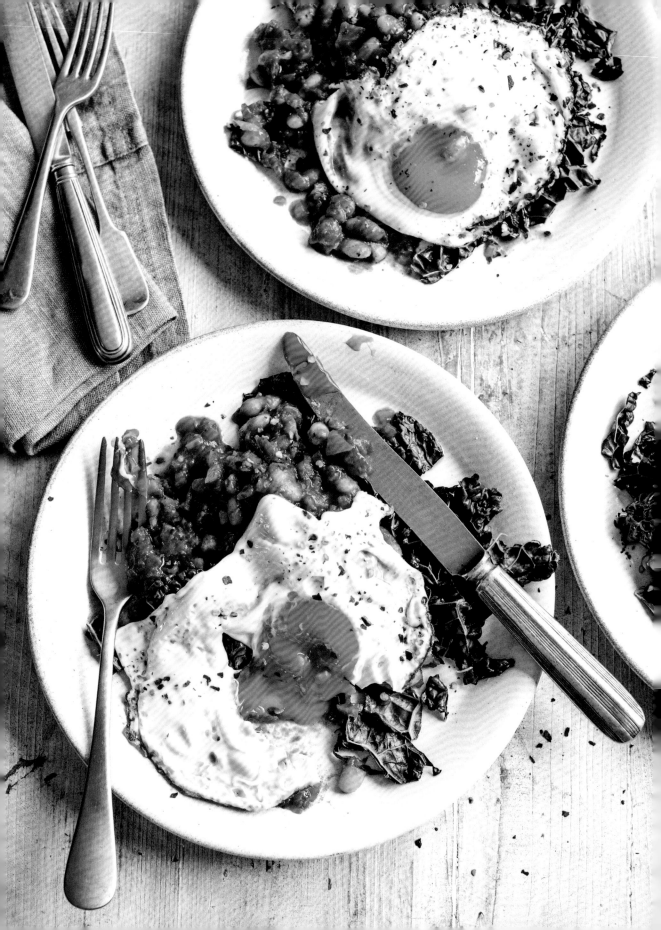

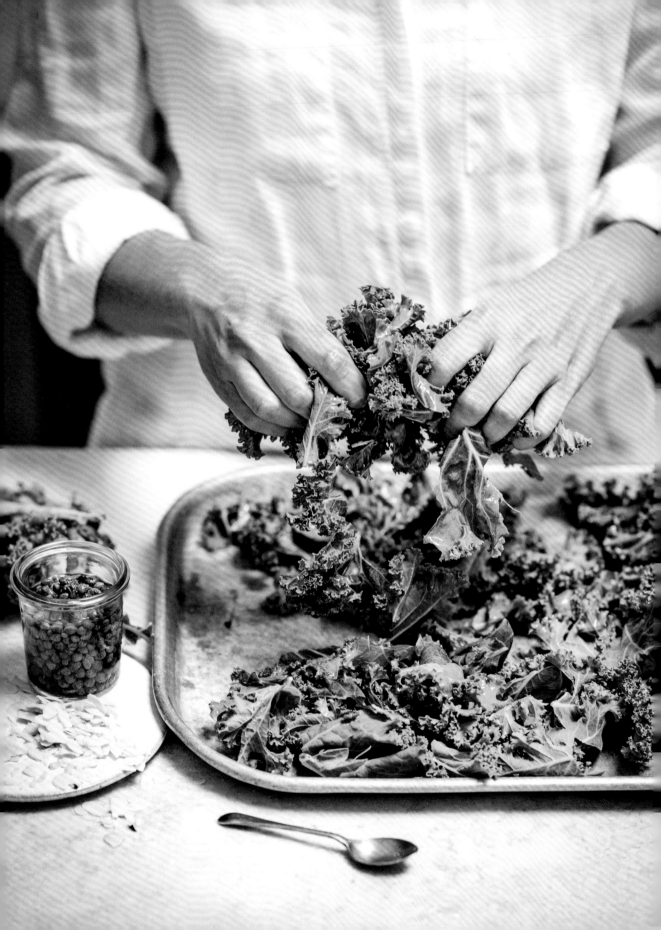

Vegetable Sides & Snacks

As you know, you are free to eat any leafy greens or non-starchy veg with a drizzle of olive oil, a small knob of butter or one of our no-count dressings (see pages 236–9), without counting the calories. We've included some examples of these here, along with more substantial veg side dishes and some easy savoury snacks for days when you have calories to spare.

PER SERVING | **232cals** | PROTEIN **6.2g** | CARBS **16.4g**

Garlicky Mashed Turnips and Cauliflower

SERVES	PREP	COOK
2	**5** mins	**30** mins

1 small turnip, peeled and chopped into 1cm cubes (approx. 400g prepared weight)
½ cauliflower, roughly chopped (approx. 350g)
2 garlic cloves, peeled and sliced
30g butter or olive oil

A pleasing mashed potato substitute, which your gut microbiome will love, thanks to the fabulous fibre and nutrients. Your microbes convert these into important substances that reduce bodily inflammation and aid weight loss.

1. Place the turnip, cauliflower and garlic in a medium saucepan, cover with boiling water and simmer, covered, for 30 minutes.

2. Drain the veg and leave to steam dry for about 1 minute.

3. Mash with the butter and a generous pinch of salt and freshly ground black pepper.

PER SERVING | **102cals** | PROTEIN **4.1g** | CARBS **5.3g**

Green Cauli Mash

SERVES	PREP	COOK
4	**5** mins	**5–7** mins

½ small cauliflower, broken into small florets
150g green veg (such as broccoli, cavolo nero or cabbage), thinly sliced
2 small leeks, trimmed and thinly sliced
2 tbsp olive oil

This scrumptious combination is a treat in itself, but also makes a tasty, low-carb side dish for mopping up sauces and stews.

1. Place the cauliflower, green veg and leeks into a large colander over a saucepan of simmering water. Cover and steam for 5–7 minutes, or until soft.

2. Transfer the veg to a bowl with the olive oil, add a generous pinch of salt and freshly ground black pepper and blitz with a stick blender until combined but retaining some texture.

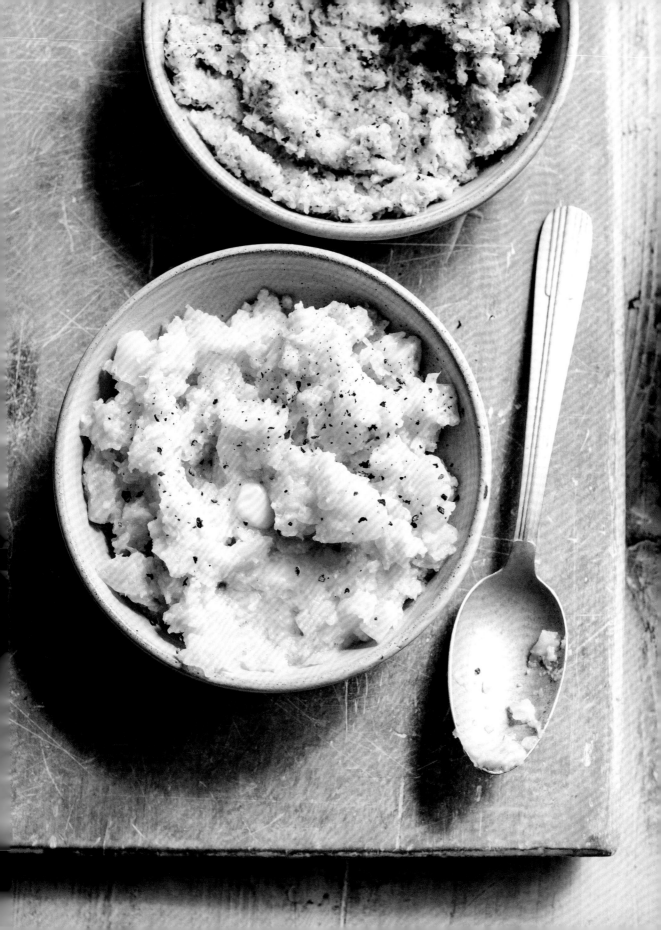

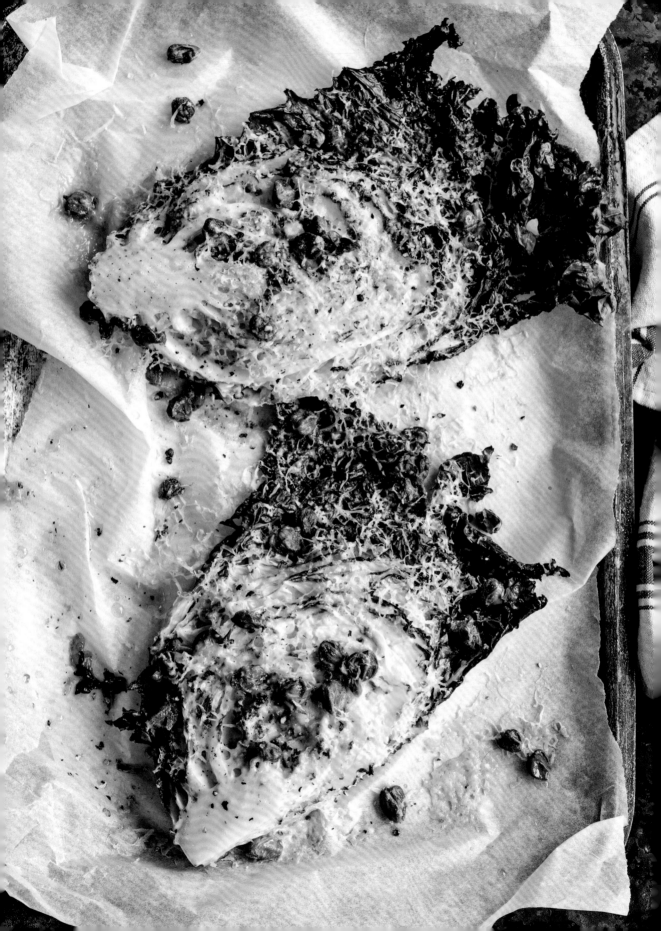

Baked Cabbage with Parmesan and Capers

SERVES	PREP	COOK
2	**5** mins	**20** mins

½ **medium savoy cabbage,
cut in half through
the core**
1 tbsp olive oil
2 tsp capers
20g Parmesan, finely grated

NON-FAST DAY
Double the portion size
and add protein top-ups
(see page 240).

When baked, cabbage takes on a slightly sweet, almost
nutty taste. With the umami flavour of Parmesan and
the sharp, zesty bursts from the capers, it is elevated
to another level!

1. Preheat the oven to 200°C/Fan 180°C/Gas 6 and line
a baking tray with baking parchment.

2. Place the cabbage wedges on the prepared baking tray,
cut-side-up, and brush with the olive oil. Season with salt
and freshly ground black pepper and roast in the oven for
15 minutes.

3. Carefully remove from the oven and press the cabbage
down with a spoon to flatten. Firmly place the capers on
top and sprinkle with the Parmesan. Return to the oven
for a further 5 minutes, until the cabbage is browned
in places and the cheese is melted.

PER SERVING | **166cals** | PROTEIN **4.4g** | CARBS **1.5g**

Crispy Kale with Anchovies and Capers

SERVES	PREP	COOK
2	**5** mins	**10** mins

2 anchovies, finely chopped
2 tbsp olive oil
150g curly kale, tough
   stalks removed
1 tbsp capers
1 level tbsp toasted flaked
   almonds (optional)

COOK'S TIP
If you choose not to include almonds, the dish will be 134cals, 3.1g protein and 1.1g carbs per serving.

When kale is cooked this way, it softens, and the exposed edges become deliciously crispy. The salty anchovies are a great flavour enhancer. They also provide a top up of health-enhancing omega-3. This would make a delicious on-the-go breakfast or brunch, if you added a couple of hard-boiled eggs.

1. Preheat the oven to 220°C/Fan 200°C/Gas 7.

2. Place the chopped anchovies and olive oil in a large bowl and mash together until mostly combined. Add the kale and use your hands to massage the oil into the leaves so that it is thoroughly coated. Spread out on a baking tray and place in the oven for 8–10 minutes.

3. Serve topped with the capers and almonds, if using.

PER SERVING | **198cals** | PROTEIN **5.9g** | CARBS **2.8g**

Kale with Garlic and Almonds

SERVES	PREP	COOK
1	**3–5** mins	**3** mins

1 tbsp olive oil
2–3 garlic cloves, peeled
 and thinly sliced
100g curly kale, tough stalk
 removed and leaves sliced
1 tbsp flaked almonds
 (optional)

A delicious and versatile side dish, this also works nicely as a quick savoury breakfast when topped with a fried egg.

1. Place the olive oil and garlic in a large frying pan over a medium heat and sauté for about 1 minute, until golden brown but not burned.

2. Add the kale, stir well and cook for about 2 minutes, until the kale is slightly softened but still retaining some bite. Season with salt and freshly ground black pepper and serve topped with the flaked almonds, if using.

PER SERVING | **163cals** | PROTEIN **5.6g** | CARBS **3.7g**

Warm Kale and Broccoli with French Dressing

SERVES	PREP	COOK
2	**2** mins	**2–3** mins

½ medium broccoli, broken into
 small florets (approx. 150g)
100g curly kale, tough stalks
 removed and leaves sliced
1 portion French Dressing
 with Tofu (see page 237)

NON-FAST DAY
Add extra protein top-ups
(see page 240) and serve
a larger portion.

Eat those greens… And add some toasted nuts or seeds or a different protein top-up for a bit of extra texture (see page 240).

1. Place the broccoli and kale in a medium saucepan and cover with boiling water. Simmer for 2–3 minutes.

2. Drain the veg and toss with the dressing. Season with salt and freshly ground pepper and serve immediately.

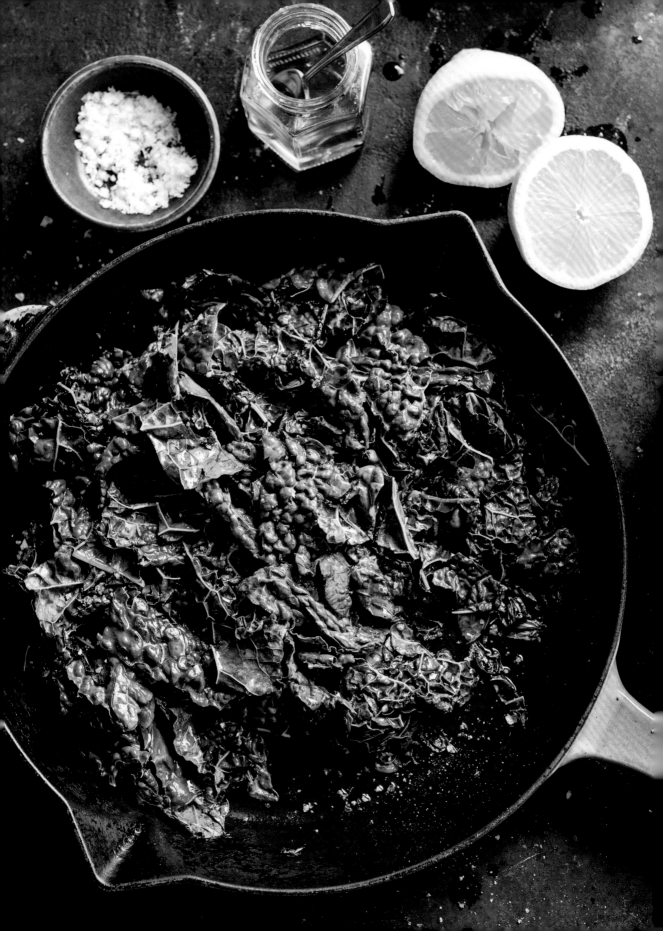

Sautéed Cavolo Nero with Lemon

SERVES | PREP | COOK
2 | **5** mins | **3** mins

**300g cavolo nero, tough
stalks removed and leaves
roughly chopped
2 tbsp olive oil
Juice of ¼ lemon**

NON-FAST DAY
Add a protein top-up
or two (see page 240),
2–3 tablespoons cooked
wholegrains and an extra
drizzle of olive oil!

With its beautiful, crinkled, dark green leaves, this is
one of my favourites as a side dish and goes with almost
anything. Adding olive oil to leafy veg helps us absorb
the nutrients.

1. Place a large frying pan over a medium heat and
add the cavolo nero and oil. Sauté for about 3 minutes,
until softened but still retaining a little bite.

2. Season with salt and freshly ground black pepper
and serve with a drizzle of lemon juice.

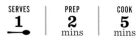

PER SERVING | **136cals** | PROTEIN **11.6g** | CARBS **11.3g**

Steamed Broccoli and Edamame Beans with Soy and Chilli

SERVES
1

PREP
2
mins

COOK
5
mins

130g tenderstem broccoli,
   trimmed
50g frozen edamame beans
1 tbsp soy sauce
Pinch of chilli flakes (optional)

NON-FAST DAY
Increase the portion
size, add a protein
top-up (see page 240)
and serve with some
non-starchy carbs.

This simple green dish pings with flavour and is high in protein and fibre, too. Add protein top-ups such as cheese, toasted nuts, cooked chicken or tofu (see page 240) for a light meal.

1. Place the broccoli in a colander set over a pan of boiling water and cover. Steam for 2 minutes. Add the edamame beans and steam for a further 2 minutes.

2. Transfer to a plate, drizzle the soy sauce all over and sprinkle with chilli flakes, if using. Season generously with freshly ground black pepper and serve.

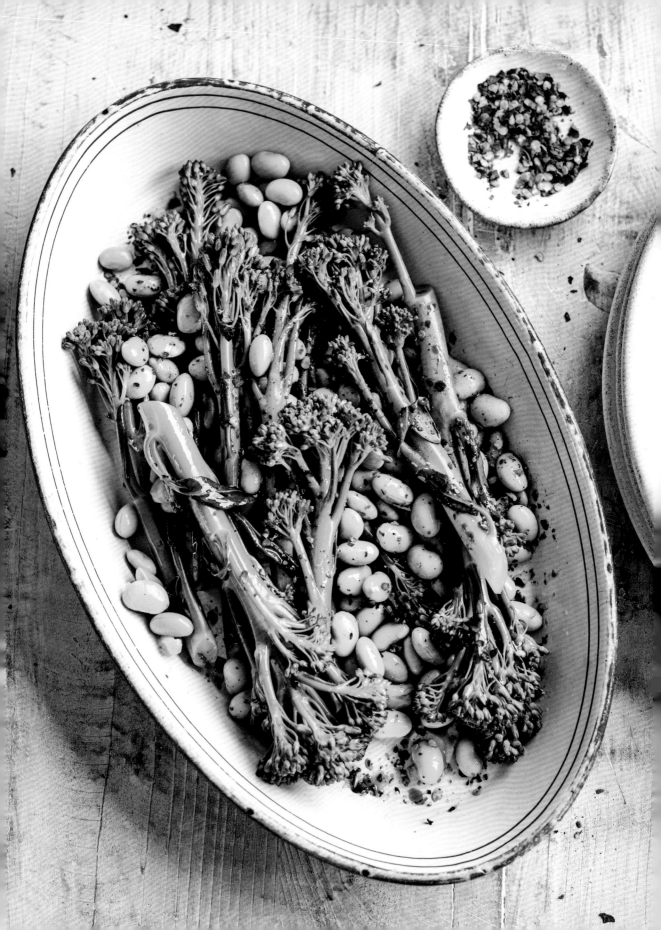

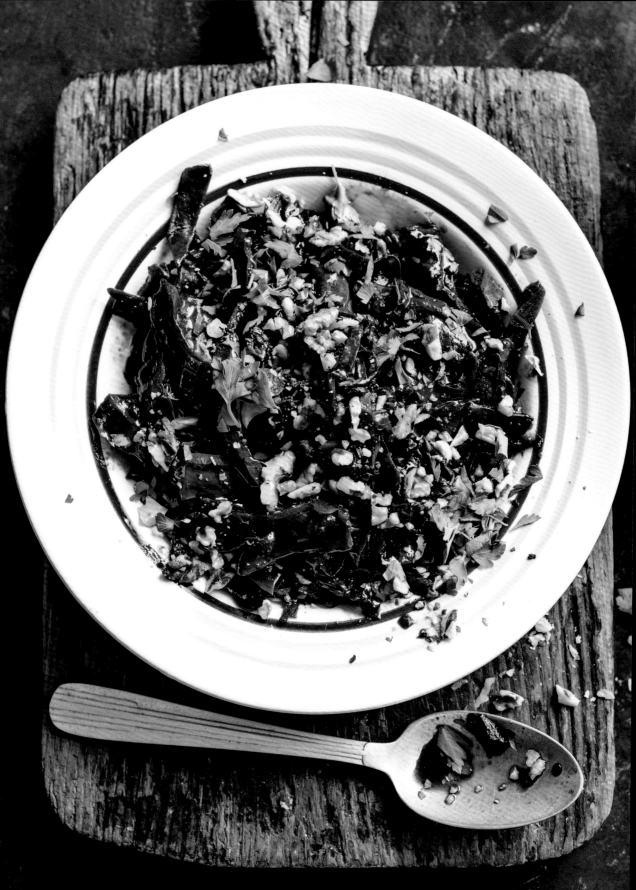

PER SERVING | **173cals** | PROTEIN **5.2g** | CARBS **9.9g**

Miso Red Cabbage

SERVES **2** | **PREP** **7–10** mins | **COOK** **15–20** mins

1 small red onion,
    peeled and sliced
½ small red cabbage
    (approx. 250g)
350ml vegetable stock
1 tbsp white miso paste
30g walnuts, roughly chopped
½ tsp chilli flakes
Small handful flat-leaf parsley,
    roughly chopped (optional)

The miso paste adds a delicious sweet and sour taste here, while the rich purple cabbage gives you a generous portion of those much-needed phytonutrients.

1. Place the onion, red cabbage and stock in a medium saucepan. Cover with a tight lid and cook over a high heat for 15–20 minutes, until the cabbage has softened and the liquid has reduced enough to coat it.

2. Stir the miso into the cabbage and taste for seasoning.

3. Serve topped with the walnuts and parsley, if using.

PER SERVING | **87cals** | PROTEIN **2.5g** | CARBS **5.6g**

Simple Coleslaw

SERVES **4** | **PREP** **10–15** mins

2 tbsp full-fat Greek yoghurt
1½ tbsp full-fat mayonnaise
1 tbsp English mustard
¼ white cabbage, finely sliced
¼ red cabbage, finely sliced

COOK'S TIP
A small handful of finely chopped rocket or spinach would make a lovely addition, if you have any in the fridge.

A coleslaw like this will sit alongside multiple different meals and will keep for up to 4 days in the fridge. The English mustard can be replaced by Dijon, if you prefer.

1. Mix the yoghurt, mayonnaise and mustard together in a large bowl.

2. Add the sliced cabbages and toss to coat thoroughly.

UNDER 200 CALORIES | PER SERVING | **109cals** | PROTEIN **4.8g** | CARBS **10g**

Oven-roasted Spiced Chickpeas

MAKES	PREP	COOK
4 portions	**5** mins	**30** mins

1 tbsp white miso paste
  (approx. 20g)
½ tsp sweet smoked paprika
1 tsp garlic granules
1 × 400g tin chickpeas,
  drained (approx. 240g
  drained weight)
1 tbsp olive oil

Scatter these on to salads, soup or stews.

1. Preheat the oven to 180°C/Fan 160°C/Gas 4 and line a baking tray with parchment paper.

2. Combine the miso paste, paprika and garlic in a medium bowl, and season with a pinch of salt and plenty of freshly ground black pepper. Add the chickpeas and olive oil and stir to coat. Spread the chickpeas on to the baking tray and roast in the oven for about 30 minutes, or until browning lightly.

3. Remove from the oven and set aside to cool.

UNDER 100 CALORIES | PER SERVING | **77cals** | PROTEIN **3.3g** | CARBS **2.3g**

Soy Roasted Seeds

MAKES	PREP	COOK
8 portions	**1–2** mins	**5–7** mins

100g pumpkin and sunflower
  seed mix (8 tablespoons)
1 tbsp soy sauce

COOK'S TIP
You can use any seeds,
but reduce the cooking
time if using small ones,
such as sesame or linseeds.

These savoury toasted seeds make a wonderful garnish for soups, salads, traybakes or even scrambled eggs, adding a healthy boost of fibre and nutrients.

1. Preheat the oven to 200°C/Fan 180°C/Gas 6 and line a baking tray with baking parchment.

2. Mix the seeds and soy sauce together in a bowl until the seeds are thoroughly coated.

3. Spread the seeds out on to the prepared tray and roast in the oven for 5–7 minutes.

4. Store in the fridge in an airtight jar. Serve 1 tablespoon per person.

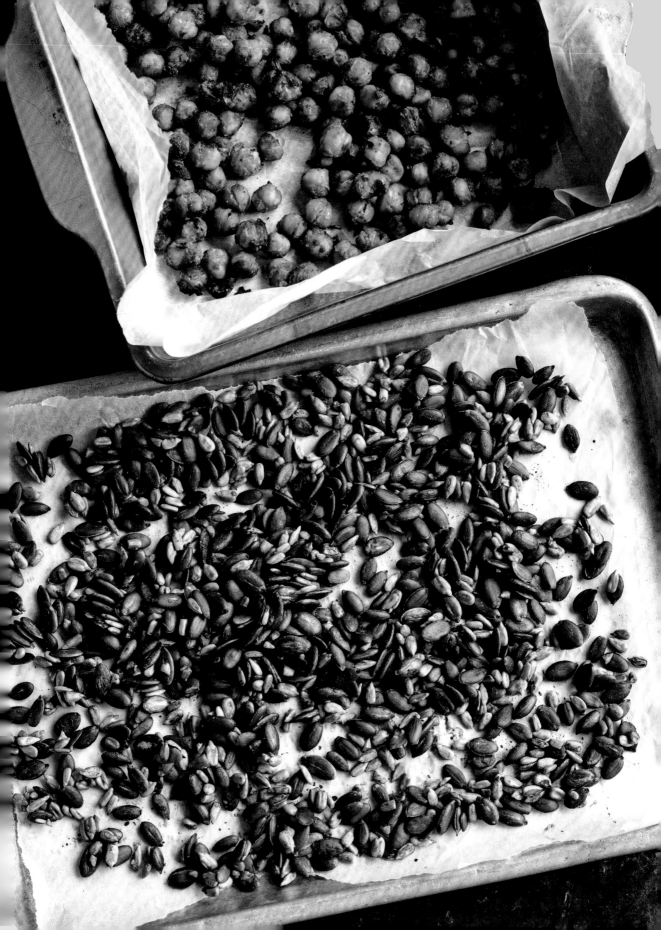

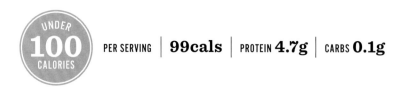

UNDER 100 CALORIES

PER SERVING | **99cals** | PROTEIN **4.7g** | CARBS **0.1g**

Salami Crisps

SERVES	PREP	COOK
2	**2** mins	**5–7** mins

8 slices good-quality salami (approx. 45g total weight)

A satisfying nibble or on-the-go snack. Best eaten on the day they are made.

1. Preheat the oven to 200°C/Fan 180°C/Gas 6 and line a baking tray with baking parchment.

2. Lay the salami on the prepared tray, leaving a bit of space between each slice. Roast in the oven for 5–7 minutes (the slices may vary in thickness so check after 5 minutes). They will start to sizzle and release their fat.

3. Remove from the oven and leave to cool on a sheet of kitchen roll.

UNDER 200 CALORIES

PER SERVING | **200cals** | PROTEIN **13.2g** | CARBS **0.9g**

Halloumi Fries

SERVES	PREP	COOK
4	**5** mins	**5–7** mins

1 tbsp olive oil
225g halloumi, cut into 8 chunky fries

A wonderfully filling addition to a meal, as well as being a great protein top-up.

1. Place the oil in a large non-stick frying pan over a high heat. When hot, add the halloumi and fry on each side until golden brown and crisp.

2. Transfer to a plate lined with kitchen paper to absorb the excess oil. Serve immediately.

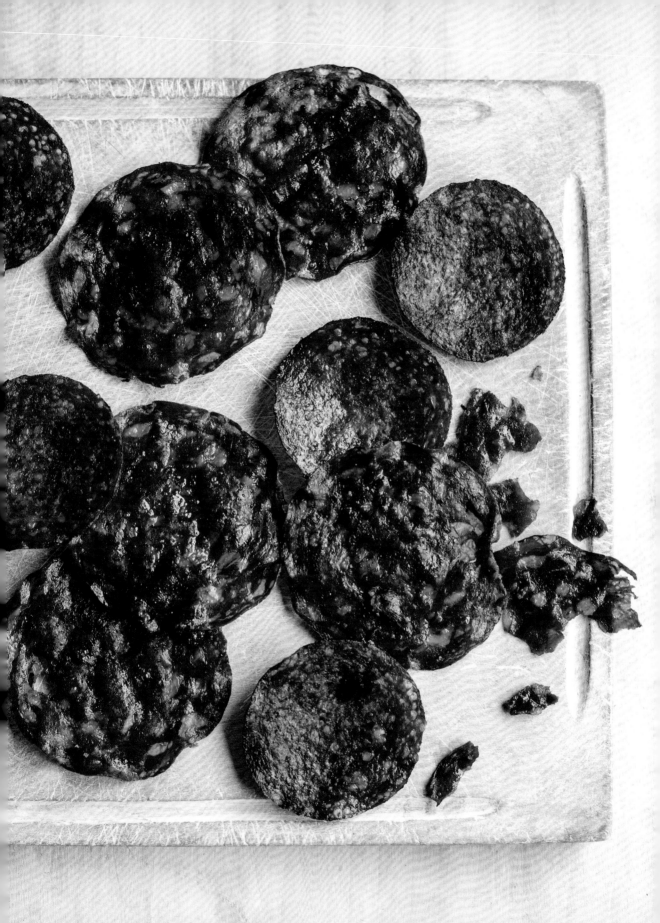

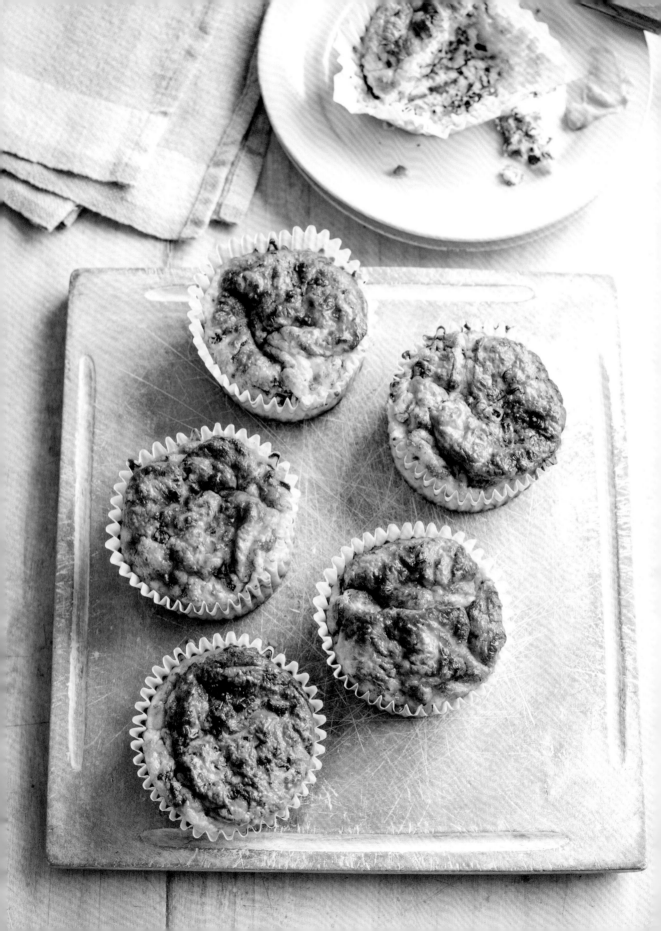

Flourless Ham, Cheese and Spinach Muffins

MAKES **6** | **PREP** **10** mins | **COOK** **15** mins

55g full-fat cream cheese
4 medium free-range eggs
30g ground almonds
¾ tsp baking powder
50g gruyere or Cheddar, grated
50g ham, roughly chopped
1 block frozen spinach (about 50g), defrosted and excess liquid squeezed out

COOK'S TIP
These muffins will keep for a couple of days refrigerated and can be frozen. They benefit from a few seconds in the microwave to freshen them up. The uncooked mixture will also keep in the fridge for 3 days so you could prepare the batter and bake them fresh as you need them.

NON-FAST DAY
Have another one!

These muffins are a great example of the keto 50:50 rule, which aims to keep carbs below 50g and protein above 50g over the day. Here there are only 0.8g carbs versus an impressive 10.9g protein, and yet each muffin only amounts to 151cals. One or two muffins are ideal for a quick, portable and filling meal.

1. Preheat the oven to 200°C/Fan 180°C/Gas 6 and line a muffin tray with 6 muffin cases (or use a silicone muffin mould).

2. Place the cream cheese, eggs, ground almonds and baking powder in a medium bowl and whisk until smooth.

3. Stir in the remaining ingredients and season with salt and freshly ground black pepper. Pour into the prepared muffin tin and bake in the oven for 15 minutes.

4. Serve warm, or leave to cool on a wire rack.

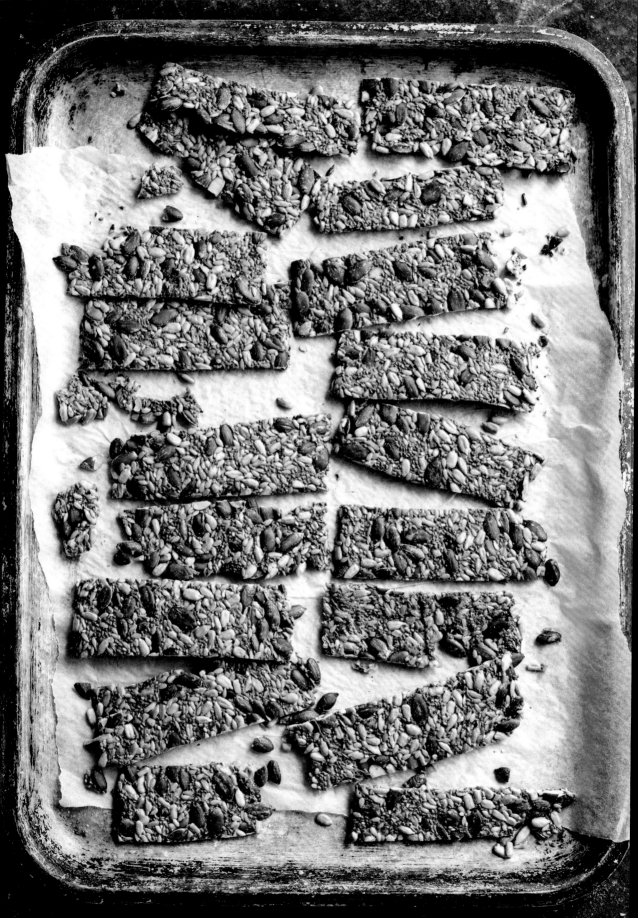

Thin Seeded Chilli Crackers

MAKES | **PREP** | **COOK**
15 | **10** mins | **15** mins

50g sunflower seeds
50g pumpkin seeds
20g linseeds
3 tbsp chia seeds (approx. 30g)
1 tbsp stoneground or
    wholegrain flour
¼ tsp cayenne pepper
¼ tsp garlic granules
½ tsp sea salt
90ml boiling hot water

NON-FAST DAY
Eat another one, or two...

These are nutritional gold dust – super-healthy, seeded, wafer-thin crackers with a hint of chilli, which are delicious on their own, or can be eaten with a dip. You could also scrunch them over a salad for added flavour and texture. An ideal snack on the go. And your gut microbiome will love them too.

1. Preheat the oven to 200°C/Fan 180°C/Gas 6 and line a baking tray no larger than 20 × 30cm with parchment paper.

2. Mix the seeds, flour and seasoning together in a large bowl. Slowly pour in the boiling water and mix well. Set aside for 10 minutes to allow the liquid to be absorbed.

3. Tip the mixture into the baking tray and, using a plastic spatula, carefully spread it out so that it is as thin as possible and fills the tray. You want the crackers to be wafer thin. Mark out 15 crackers with the tip of a knife – this will help to snap them evenly when they are cooked. Bake in the oven for 12–15 minutes, or until the seeds are golden.

4. Store in an airtight container.

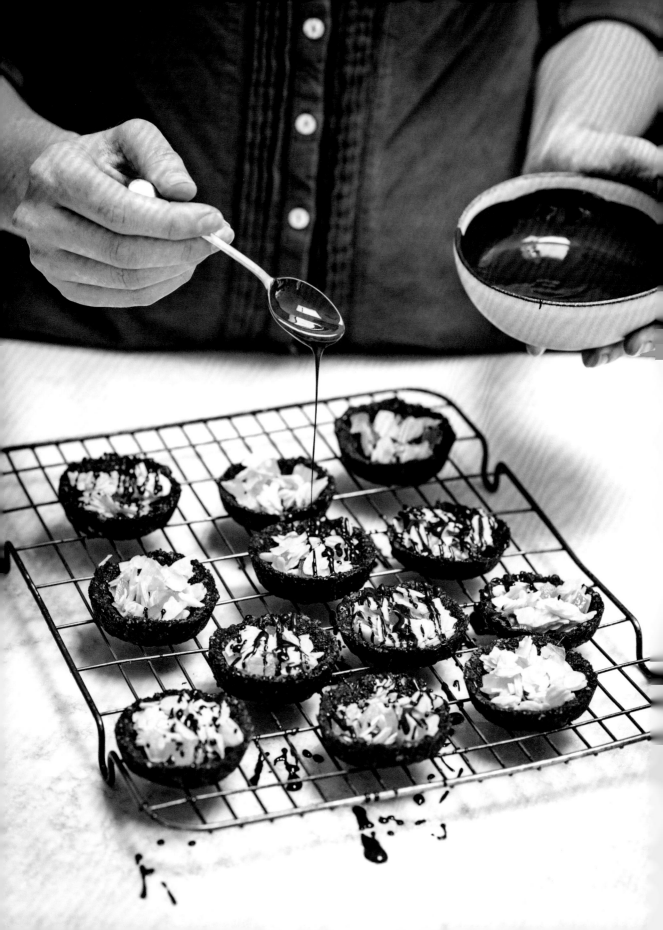

Occasional Treats

These are as keto-friendly as you can get. The trick when it comes to reducing sugar spikes is to eat treats and desserts at the end of a savoury meal, rather than on an empty stomach. You won't feel deprived!

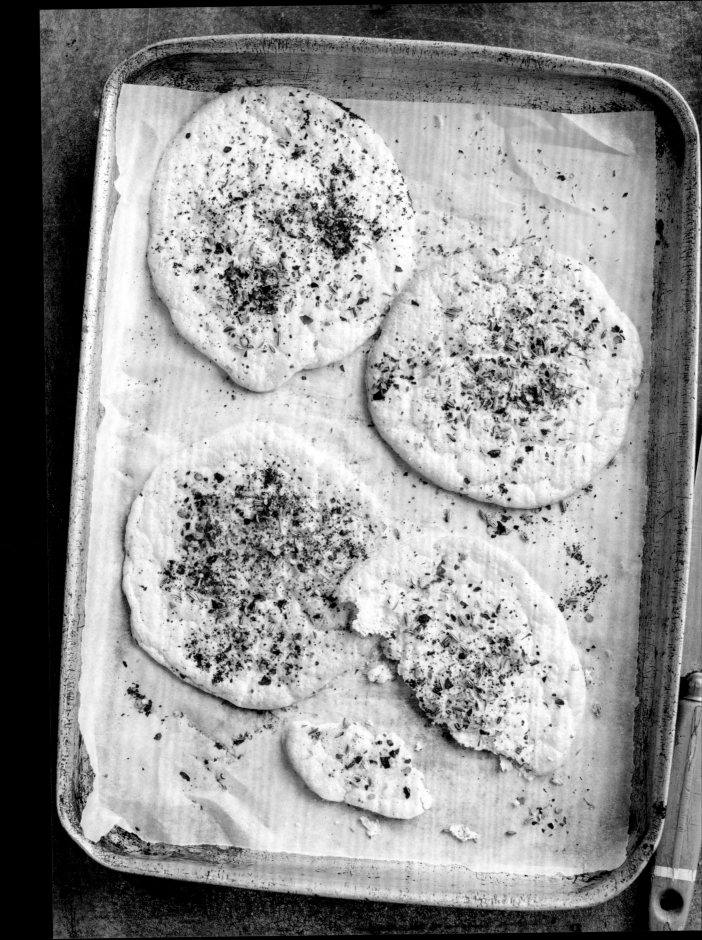

Cloud Bread

MAKES | **PREP** | **COOK**
4 | **10** mins | **15** mins

2 medium free-range eggs,
   separated
35g full-fat cream cheese
Pinch of cream of tartar

If you are missing bread, this offers an ideal keto solution. Light and soft, it is great for small sandwiches, or to replace burger buns. You could also use it as a base for an open sandwich. For variety, try flavouring the mixture with spices and dried herbs.

1. Preheat the oven to 150°C/Fan 130°C/Gas 3 and line a baking tray with baking parchment. Lightly oil the parchment paper with a flavourless oil such as sunflower or groundnut oil.

2. Place the egg whites in a clean bowl and whisk with an electric beater for about 3 minutes, until very stiff.

3. Place the egg yolks, cream cheese, cream of tartar and a generous pinch of salt and freshly ground black pepper into another bowl. Whisk with an electric beater for about 1 minute, until completely smooth.

4. Using a spatula, gently fold the egg whites into the cream cheese mixture until thoroughly mixed. Spoon four circles of the mixture onto the prepared baking tray and cook in the oven for 15 minutes, until firm and golden brown.

5. Leave to cool completely before removing from the baking parchment.

PER SERVING | **245cals** | PROTEIN **9.6g** | CARBS **2.7g**

Instant Mug Bread

SERVES	PREP	COOK
2	**5** mins	**2** mins

1 level tbsp salted butter
1 heaped tbsp flaxseed
3 heaped tbsp ground almonds
1 level tbsp seeds of your choice
   (such as pumpkin, sunflower
   or linseed)
1 tsp baking powder
1 small free-range egg

COOK'S TIP

Don't be disconcerted
if you find a few holes in
the bread when you turn
it out of the mug. It is best
eaten on the same day,
although you can slice
it and freeze any extra
portions for toast.

This remarkable high-protein keto bread is cooked
in the microwave in a mug in less than 5 minutes.
It can be used as a breakfast muffin to enjoy with
scrambled eggs, as the base of an open sandwich,
or with a bowl of soup or even alongside a stew
to mop up juices. It also makes satisfying toast.

1. Place the butter in a mug and melt in the microwave
for 8–10 seconds. Swirl it around the sides of the mug
to grease it.

2. Add the rest of the ingredients and a pinch of salt and
mix vigorously to make sure everything is well combined.
Cook in the microwave for about 60–90 seconds.

3. Remove from the microwave and tap the top – if it's
firm and springy, it's ready. If it's soft, return it to the
microwave for another 10 seconds at a time, until firm.

4. Turn it upside down, tap to remove it from the mug,
and place on a wire rack to cool. Cut into circular slices
to serve.

Pears with Cardamom, Walnuts and Chocolate

SERVES	PREP	COOK
4	**10** mins	**35** mins

4 firm pears, halved
   lengthways and core
   removed (approx. 600–700g
   prepared weight)
½ tsp ground cardamom
60g walnuts, roughly chopped
40g dark chocolate
   (70% or more), chopped
   into small pieces

COOK'S TIP
If you can't find
ground cardamom
you can use cinnamon.

One of my favourite and easy go-to puddings. The cardamom adds a hint of exotic flavour to the juicy, baked pear, which sets off the melted dark chocolate and roasted walnuts nicely.

1. Preheat the oven to 190°C/Fan 170°C/Gas 5.

2. Place the pears in a baking dish, cut-side-up and add 150ml water. Scatter the cardamom over and bake in the oven for 30 minutes.

3. Remove from the oven, scatter with the nuts and chocolate and return to the oven for a final 5 minutes, until the chocolate has melted.

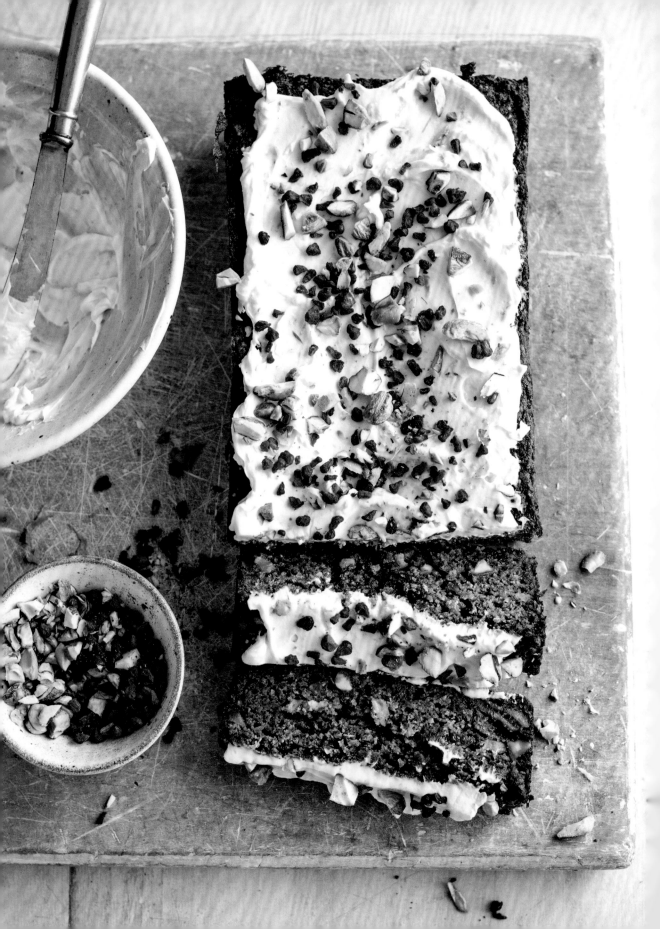

Persian Love Cake

SERVES	PREP	COOK
8	**30** mins	**30** mins

100g dried figs, finely chopped
60g coconut oil or butter
2 medium free-range eggs
60g shelled pistachio nuts,
　roughly chopped
2 medium oranges, zested
　and juiced
100g ground almonds
1 tsp ground cinnamon
1 tsp ground cardamom
1 tsp bicarbonate of soda
2 tbsp freeze-dried raspberries
1 tbsp cider vinegar

For the icing:
60g cream cheese
1 tsp honey
1 tsp lemon zest

COOK'S TIP
This freezes well (so you
don't need to eat it all
at once, as Michael is
frequently tempted to do).
You could use a loaf tin
liner if you have one.

Loosely based on a Persian Love Cake, this enchantingly
exotic concoction lives up to its name. Not sure I do it
justice, but it certainly goes down well, with its tangy,
orange-flavoured topping, and rich, nutty base. High in
protein and nutrients, it has no added sugar, is low carb
and feels like a real treat... Enjoy!

1. Preheat the oven to 180°C/Fan 160°C/Gas 4. Line
the base of a 20 x 10cm loaf tin with parchment paper.

2. Place the figs, coconut oil and eggs in a bowl and blitz
with a stick blender for about 1 minute, until creamy
but retaining some texture.

3. Stir in 40g of the pistachios, the orange juice, half the
orange zest, the ground almonds, cinnamon, cardamom,
bicarbonate of soda, half the dried raspberries and a
generous pinch of salt. Mix well, then add the cider
vinegar and mix again.

4. Pour the mixture into the loaf tin and bake for about
30 minutes, until cooked through and a skewer inserted
into the centre comes out clean. Turn out of the tin and
leave to cool on a wire rack.

5. To make the topping, mix the remaining orange zest
with the cream cheese, honey and lemon zest in a small
bowl. Spread it on to the cooled cake, then sprinkle the
remaining chopped pistachios and dried raspberries
on top.

PER SERVING | **160cals** | PROTEIN **7.1g** | CARBS **4.1g**

Pear and Rosemary Muffins

MAKES	PREP	COOK
6	**10** mins	**15** mins

85g ground almonds
1 sprig of rosemary, leaves
    picked and finely chopped
1 tsp baking powder
1 tbsp coconut oil (approx. 15g)
75g full-fat Greek yoghurt
1 tsp honey
2 medium free-range eggs
½ × 415g tin pears in juice,
    drained and finely chopped
    (115g drained weight)

Fruit-sweetened muffins with the delicate flavour of rosemary. Satisfyingly filling yet low in carbs.

1. Preheat the oven to 200°C/Fan 180°C/Gas 6 and line a muffin tray with six cases.

2. Mix the dry ingredients together in a medium bowl.

3. Place the coconut oil in another medium bowl and melt in the microwave for a few seconds. Add the yoghurt, honey, a pinch of salt and the eggs. Whisk to combine.

4. Add the dry ingredients to the wet ingredients and mix well. Gently fold in the chopped pears and spoon the mixture into the muffin cases. Bake for 15 minutes, or until golden.

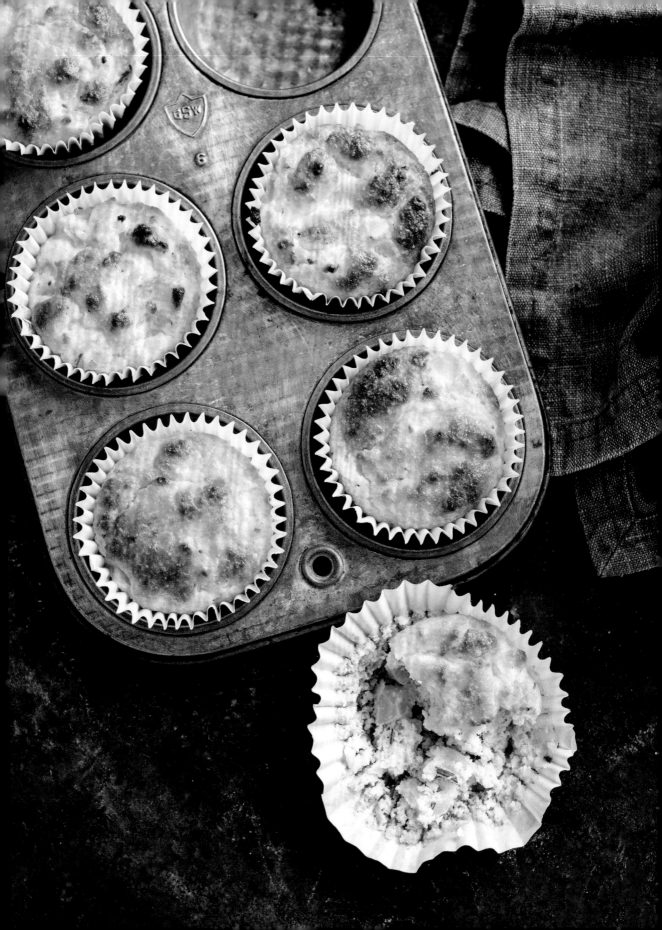

Chocolate Florentines

SERVES	PREP	COOK
12	**15** mins	**10** mins

1 tbsp coconut oil,
   plus extra for greasing
1 ripe small banana
   (approx. 65g peeled weight),
   peeled and mashed
40g rolled oats
40g desiccated coconut
1 tbsp cocoa powder
2 balls of stem ginger
   (approx. 20g), diced
1 tbsp ginger syrup
50g flaked almonds,
   roughly chopped
60g dark chocolate
   (70% or more)

Another healthy low-carb indulgence. Ideal for
a celebration!

1. Preheat the oven to 170°C/Fan 150°C/Gas 3 and
grease a 12-hole cupcake tray with a little coconut oil.
Line a baking tray with parchment paper.

2. Place the coconut oil in a bowl and melt in the
microwave for a few seconds. Add the mashed banana,
rolled oats, desiccated coconut and cocoa powder and
mix well.

3. Using a dessert spoon, divide the mixture between
the holes of the cupcake tray and press it into the base
and sides to line them. Bake in the oven for 5 minutes.

4. Meanwhile, mix the stem ginger, syrup and flaked
almonds together in a small bowl, so the almonds are
well coated.

5. Remove the tray from the oven and, using a teaspoon,
spread the sticky almond mixture into the bases. Return
to the oven for about 5 minutes, or until the nuts are
slightly golden in places. Remove from the oven and
set aside to cool.

6. Melt the chocolate in the microwave or using a bain
marie. Remove the biscuits from the tray and dip each
one in the chocolate to coat the base (or drizzle chocolate
over the top). Place them on the prepared baking tray
to set. Store in the fridge or a cool place.

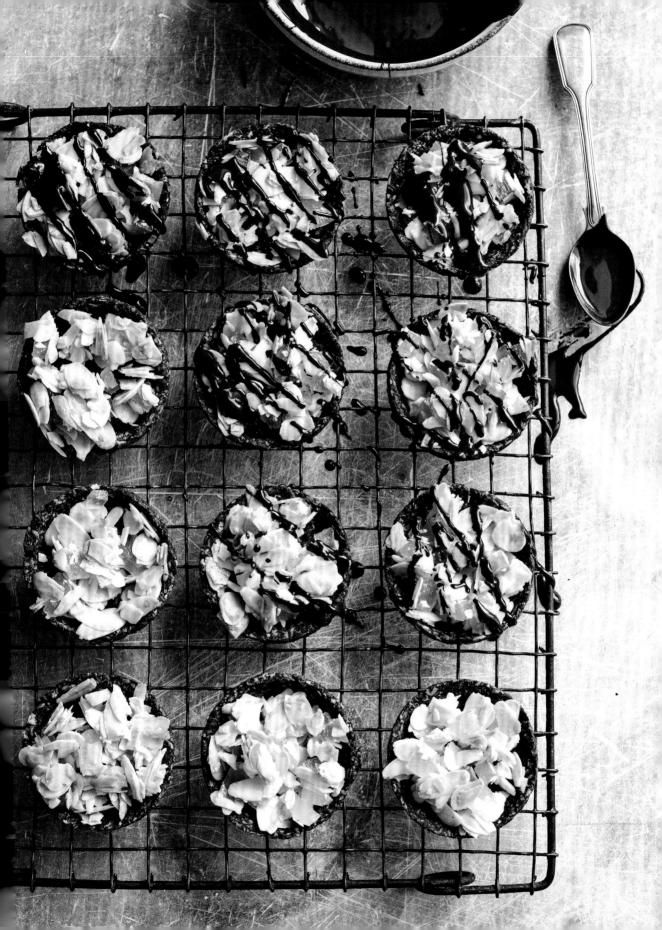

PER SERVING | **77cals** | PROTEIN **3.3g** | CARBS **5.3g**

Banana and Pistachio Pancakes

MAKES	PREP	COOK
8	**10** mins	**10** mins

2 medium bananas, peeled
    (approx. 200g peeled weight)
50g ground almonds
2 medium free-range eggs
1 tsp vanilla extract
50g shelled pistachios,
    roughly chopped
Small knob of butter or 1 tsp oil
1 tbsp freeze-dried raspberries

COOK'S TIP
These should resemble
Scotch pancakes
(drop scones).

These exotic-looking mini pancakes, with a Middle Eastern feel to them thanks to the green pistachio nuts and the brightly coloured raspberry pieces, taste every bit as good as they look.

1. Mash the bananas in a medium bowl. Add the ground almonds, eggs, vanilla extract and a pinch of salt and whisk together.

2. Stir in half of the pistachios and add a little water, if the mixture is dry rather than gloopy.

3. Place the butter or oil in a non-stick frying pan over a medium heat. When hot, pour in the mixture a tablespoon at a time and cook 3 or 4 together for 1–2 minutes, until golden, being careful not to burn them. They are ready to turn when small bubbles are visible on the surface.

4. Scatter with some of the remaining pistachios and dried raspberries, then flip with a spatula and cook for another minute or more. Set aside and repeat with the remaining batter.

5. Pile the pancakes on to a plate and serve with crème fraîche (1 tablespoon is 45cals) or fresh raspberries.

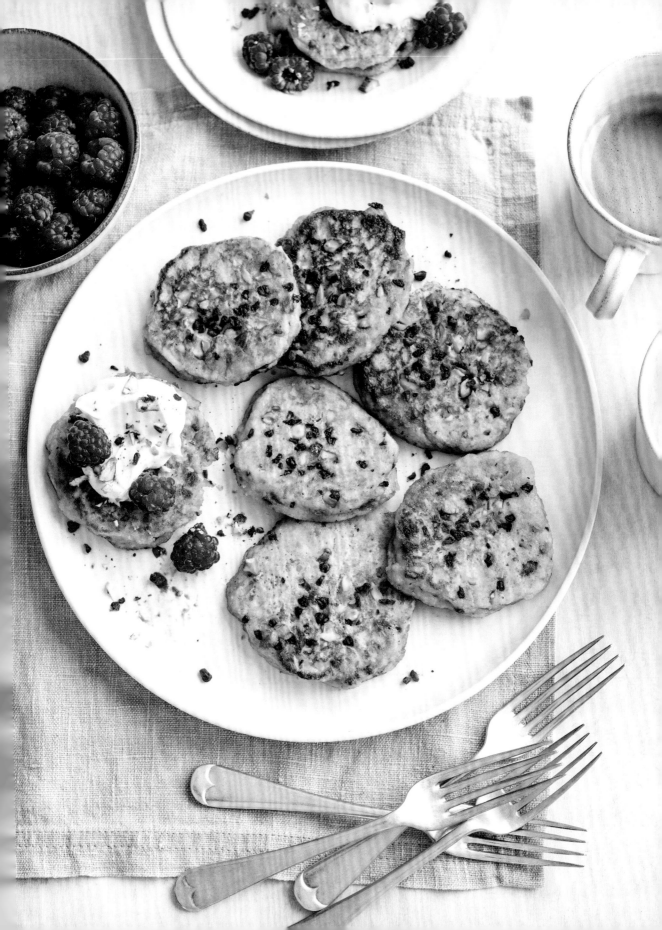

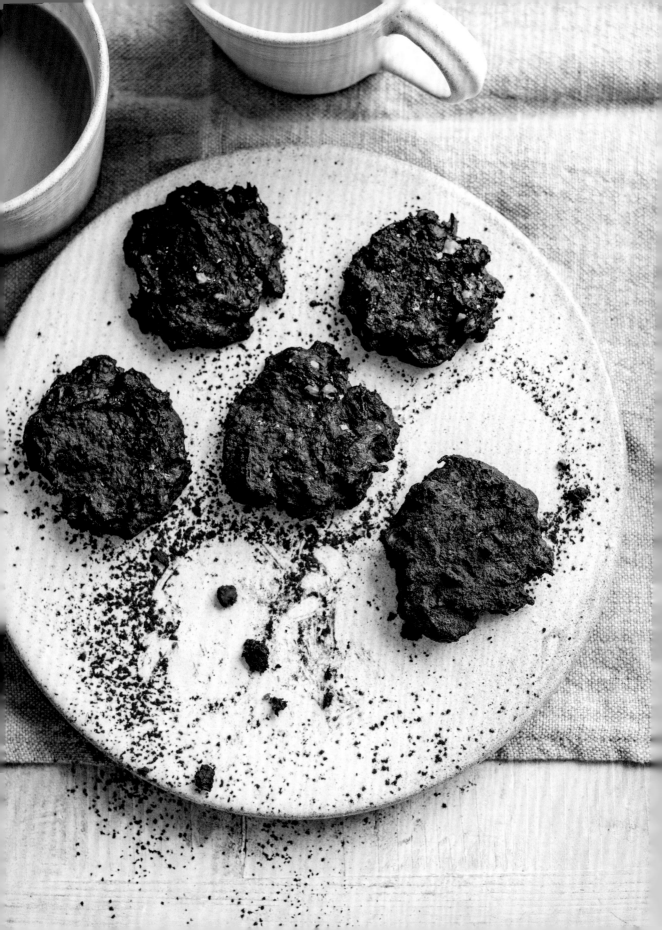

Chocolate Peanut Butter Cookies

SERVES	PREP	COOK
6	**5** mins	**10** mins

1 good-sized ripe banana,
  peeled and mashed (approx.
  100g prepared weight)
2 level tbsp crunchy or smooth
  peanut butter (approx. 30g)
2 level tbsp cocoa powder

A cracking good keto cookie which is slightly soft
in the middle, incredibly easy to make and a great
way to use up a ripe banana.

1. Preheat the oven to 200°C/Fan 180°C/Gas 6 and
line a baking tray with baking parchment.

2. Mix all the ingredients in a medium bowl with
a pinch of salt.

3. Dollop 6 cookies onto the tray and cook for about
12 minutes, or until firm to touch.

4. Allow to cool before removing from the tray.

PER SERVING | **133cals** | PROTEIN **3g** | CARBS **10.7g**

No-added-sugar Dark Chocolate Cookies

MAKES	PREP	COOK
12	**25** mins	**15** mins

3 tbsp coconut oil, melted
6 level tbsp ground almonds
6 level tbsp rolled oats
2 medium free-range
    egg whites
Generous pinch of salt
¼–½ tsp cinnamon, to taste
12 soft dates, finely diced
    (approx. 90g total weight)
1 tbsp cocoa
50g dark chocolate
    (70% or more), chopped
    into small pieces

Chocolate biscuits made with tablespoon measures and mixed in one bowl with a wooden spoon. So easy! Save a few in a bag in the freezer so you don't overdo it, as they are quite moreish.

1. Preheat the oven to 190°C/Fan 170°C/Gas 5 and line a large baking tray with parchment paper.

2. Place all the ingredients in a large bowl and mix vigorously with a wooden spoon. Add a tablespoon of water to loosen, if necessary.

3. Dollop small tablespoonfuls of mixture onto the paper, pressing down slightly to flatten. Bake in the oven for 15–20 minutes, until the cookies are starting to brown very slightly.

4. Remove from the oven and leave to cool on a wire rack.

Easy Strawberry, Mint and Peach Salad

SERVES
1

PREP
5
mins

½ × 415g tin peaches in juice
  (not syrup!), drained and
  sliced (approx. 125g
  drained weight)
100g strawberries, sliced
Small handful of mint
  leaves, sliced
2 tbsp full-fat Greek yoghurt

We have really begun to enjoy tinned peaches in juice (rather than in syrup, which is far higher in sugar). Fruit contains lots of anti-inflammatory phytonutrients, but it also contains sugar so it is best eaten with, or straight after, a meal to reduce blood sugar spikes. Strawberries add extra sweetness, which interestingly comes mostly from a sugar aroma rather than actual sugar.

1. Arrange the peaches and strawberries in a bowl, scatter the mint leaves over and top with the yoghurt.

PER SERVING | **86cals** | PROTEIN **1g** | CARBS **8.7g**

Chocolate Hazelnut Thins

SERVES	PREP	COOK
6	**5** mins	**5** mins

75g dark chocolate
(70% or more)
1 heaped tbsp chopped
toasted hazelnuts
Pinch of chilli flakes
or ground cardamom
(or seeds from 2 pods)
(optional)
½ tbsp freeze-dried
raspberries

COOK'S TIP

You can toast your own chopped hazelnuts in a dry frying pan over a medium heat, shaking and turning frequently, for about 2 minutes, until golden brown.

These tasty, nutty thins take 5 minutes to prepare before a meal and are ready to nibble 30 minutes later. For a delicious instant pudding you can scatter them on top of a couple of tinned pears and serve with a dollop of full-fat Greek yoghurt.

1. Line a baking tray with parchment paper.

2. Break up the chocolate and melt in a heatproof bowl set over a pan of simmering water, or in the microwave.

3. Pour the chocolate onto the prepared tray and use a spatula to spread thinly (about 2–3mm).

4. Scatter the hazelnuts, chilli or cardamom, if using, and the dried raspberries onto the chocolate while it is still soft, then place in the freezer to set (you can also set in the fridge but it will take longer).

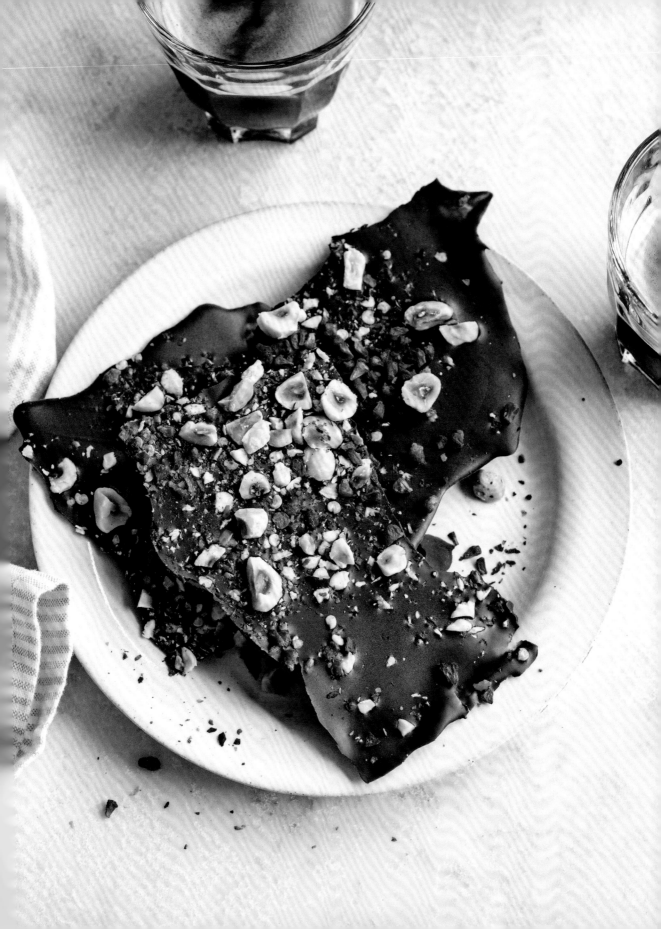

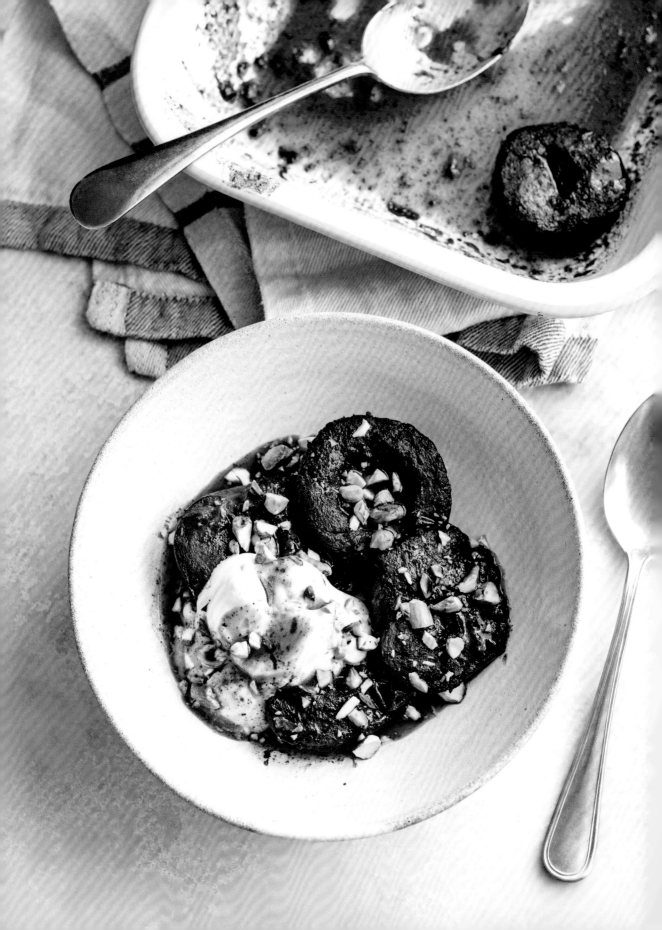

Baked Plums with Pistachios and Vanilla Yoghurt

SERVES	PREP	COOK
2	**5** mins	**25** mins

4 large plums, halved and
    destoned (approx. 300g
    total weight)
1 tbsp coconut oil
1 tsp ground cinnamon
    or ginger
2 tbsp shelled pistachios,
    roughly chopped
50g full-fat Greek yoghurt
1 tbsp vanilla extract

*Juicy baked plums with green pistachios –
a glorious summer indulgence.*

1. Preheat the oven to 180°C/Fan 160°C/Gas 4.

2. Place the plums cut-side-up in a small baking dish.
Spread with the coconut oil and sprinkle over the
cinnamon or ginger.

3. Add 2 tablespoons of water to the dish and bake in
the oven for 15 minutes, until the plums are starting
to brown slightly.

4. Carefully remove from the oven, scatter over the
nuts and return to the oven for a further 10 minutes,
until the nuts are slightly browned and the plums
are softening and scorched in places.

5. Meanwhile, combine the yoghurt and vanilla in
a small bowl and dollop over the plums to serve.

PER SERVING | **257cals** | PROTEIN **8.9g** | CARBS **11.9g**

Instant Rhubarb Pudding with Diced Stem Ginger

SERVES | PREP | COOK
2 | **10** mins | **3** mins

1 tbsp coconut oil
50g fresh rhubarb, diced
4 level tbsp ground almonds (approx. 40g)
1 tsp baking powder
1 tsp vanilla extract
2 balls stem ginger from a jar, drained and finely diced
1 medium free-range egg, beaten
2–3 small drops red food colouring (optional)

COOK'S TIP

You could dice 500g rhubarb to make stewed rhubarb, cooking it with ½ teaspoon honey in the microwave or a small pan with a dash of water until soft. High in healthy phytonutrients, this doesn't need counting. Avoid getting the red food colouring on you as it can stain.

I love an instant pudding – and whisked together in a mug and heated in the microwave is about as instant as you can get. Rhubarb is quite tart, so it works well with a bit of sweetness from the diced stem ginger. The two drops of natural colouring are just a bit of fun to enhance the pinkness of the rhubarb which fades on cooking. You might also like to dollop a tablespoon of creamy Greek yoghurt on top (see page 240 for calories).

1. Place the coconut oil and diced rhubarb in a large microwave-safe cup and cook in the microwave for 1 minute.

2. Mix in the ground almonds, baking powder, a pinch of salt, the vanilla extract and diced ginger. Stir in the egg and colouring, if using, and mix together vigorously.

3. Return the cup to the microwave for 90 seconds. Tap the top and, if it is firm, set it aside to cool a little before turning it out. If it is not firm, return it to the microwave and cook for another 10 seconds at a time until cooked.

Stewed Apple with Nuts and Cinnamon

SERVES **2** | **PREP** **15** mins | **COOK** **10** mins

2 medium Bramley apples,
  cored, not peeled, and cut
  into smallish chunks
  (approx. 225g total weight)
1 tsp ground cinnamon
20g raisins
4 tbsp full-fat Greek yoghurt
50g flaked almonds, toasted

COOK'S TIP
You can keep this in
the fridge for several
days, or freeze for later
if there is any left over.

A homely and comforting pudding. By not peeling
the apples, not only do you save time, you also benefit
from the extra nutrients and fibre in the skin.

1. Place the apple in a saucepan, add a splash of water,
cover with a lid and warm over a medium heat. Check
after 5 minutes to make sure it doesn't burn – it's ready
when the apple is turning fluffy and the chunks are soft
(about 10 minutes).

2. Remove from the heat and stir in the cinnamon
and raisins.

3. Serve warm or cold with the yoghurt and flaked almonds.

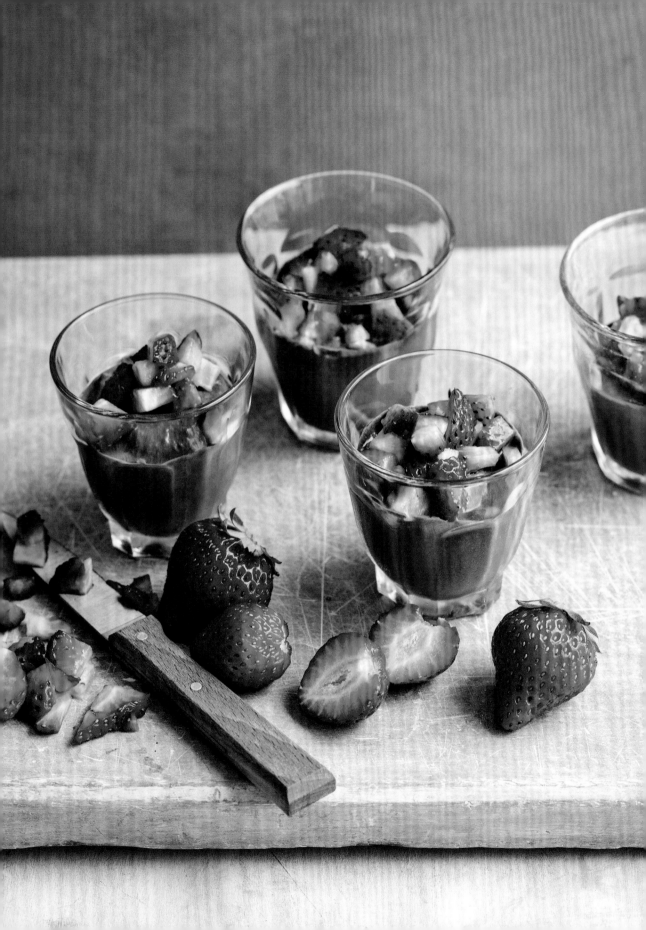

Mocha Mousse Pots with Strawberries

SERVES | PREP
4 | **12–15** mins

60g dark chocolate
   (70% or more)
1 tbsp instant coffee
   (made with ½ tsp
   instant coffee granules)
120g full-fat Greek yoghurt
2 medium free-range
   egg whites
60g strawberries, chopped

COOK'S TIP
Remember to remove
the chocolate from the
heat as soon as it has
softened as it can turn
crumbly when over-cooked.

With only three main ingredients, these can be
whipped up in a matter of minutes. Topped with some
strawberries, they make the perfect summer dessert.

1. Melt the chocolate in a heatproof bowl set over a pan
of simmering water, or in the microwave.

2. Allow to cool a little, then stir in the coffee. Add the
yoghurt and beat until thoroughly combined.

3. In a separate bowl, whisk the egg whites until very stiff.
Fold a spoon of the egg white into the chocolate mixture
to loosen, then gently fold in the rest, until combined.

4. Divide between four small glasses and refrigerate for a
few hours or overnight. Top with the strawberries to serve.

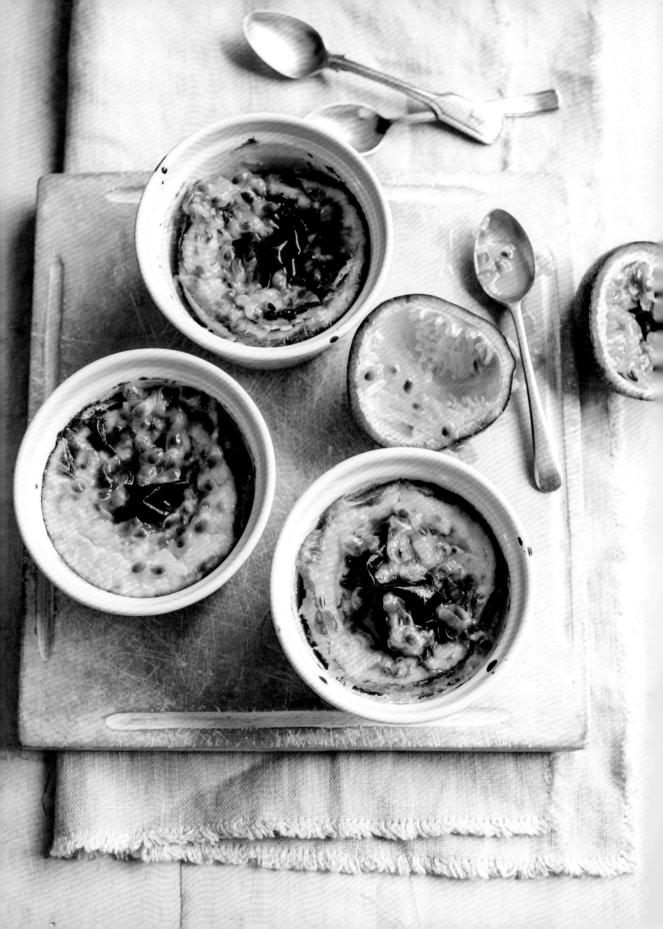

Peach and Vanilla Mini Basque Cheesecakes

SERVES	PREP	COOK
6	**5–7** mins	**20** mins

Coconut oil, for greasing
160g full-fat cream cheese
½ × 415g tin peaches in
　juice, drained (125g
　drained weight)
½ tbsp vanilla extract
1 medium free-range egg
2 medium free-range egg yolks
1 large or 2 small passionfruit

COOK'S TIP

If you don't have ramekin dishes you can use a muffin tin lined with 6 muffin cases. Keep any leftovers in the fridge for up to 3 days.

These delightful little cheesecakes come out of the oven with a deep golden, almost burnt-looking surface and are light and delicate inside. Spices, such as ground cardamom or cinnamon, would make a lovely addition.

1. Preheat the oven to 240°C/Fan 220°C/Gas 9 and grease 6 × 20cm ramekins with a little coconut oil.

2. Place the cream cheese, peaches, vanilla extract, egg and egg yolks in a jug and blitz with a stick blender until smooth.

3. Pour into the ramekin dishes and bake in the oven for 20 minutes, or until the tops are golden brown. Allow to cool.

4. Cut a passionfruit in half and scrape out the seeds with a teaspoon. Spoon over the cheesecakes to serve.

PER SERVING | **193cals** | PROTEIN **3.7g** | CARBS **9g**

Pear and Chocolate Raspberry Crumble

SERVES	PREP	COOK
4	**5** mins	**10** mins

100g fresh or frozen
    raspberries
2 tinned pear halves,
    drained and sliced
25g dark chocolate,
    cut into small chunks
25g desiccated coconut
50g broken walnuts
2 tbsp full-fat Greek yoghurt

COOK'S TIP
The remaining pears in
the tin will keep in the
fridge for several days.
You can use them for
breakfast – top half a
pear with a tablespoon
of Greek yoghurt and a
tablespoon of walnuts.

NON-FAST DAY
Add extra nuts and yoghurt.

A classic fruit combination with a little
indulgence and plenty of fibre.

1. Preheat the oven 190°C/Fan 170°C/Gas 5.

2. Divide the raspberries between four ramekins
and top each pile of berries with pear.

3. Scatter the chocolate chunks, coconut and walnuts
over the tops and bake in the oven for 8 minutes,
until warmed through and the nuts are just toasted.

4. Serve with the yoghurt alongside.

Chocolate and Fruit Chia Yoghurt Pot

SERVES
2

PREP
5
mins

100g full-fat Greek yoghurt
100ml full-fat milk
1 level tbsp unsweetened
   cocoa powder
20g chia seeds
½ tinned pear (in juice),
   finely chopped
50g fresh or frozen raspberries

COOK'S TIP
These chocolate pots
can be made ahead
and kept in the fridge
to enjoy after a meal.

NON-FAST DAY
Add some toasted
chopped nuts.

This works as a treat after a meal, or indeed as a special breakfast. Chia is a versatile 'superfood' worth getting to know. Here it adds creaminess.

1. Place the yoghurt, milk, cocoa powder and chia seeds in a medium bowl and whisk until completely combined.

2. Stir in the pear and half the raspberries.

3. Divide between two small bowls or jars, scatter with the remaining raspberries and leave in the fridge to set for 3 hours. If leaving them overnight you may need a dash of milk or water to loosen them to a creamy texture.

PER SERVING | **95cals** | PROTEIN **6.2g** | CARBS **8.9g**

Mango and Lime Semifreddo

SERVES **6** | PREP **10–15** mins

250g full-fat Greek yoghurt
Zest of 1 lime
1 tbsp vanilla extract
2 medium free-range
 eggs, separated
1 × 425g tin mangoes in juice,
 drained and blitzed until
 smooth (approx. 230g
 drained weight)

A simple but indulgent frozen dessert. A very ripe fresh mango could be used here, but the beauty of using tinned is that you can have it on hand, ready to pull together whenever you fancy.

1. Line a 450g loaf tin with 2 large sheets of clingfilm, leaving the excess hanging over the sides of the tin.

2. Place the yoghurt, lime zest, vanilla and egg yolks in a bowl and whisk until smooth. Stir in three quarters of the blitzed mango.

3. Place the egg whites in a separate bowl and whisk until very stiff.

4. Gently fold the egg whites into the yoghurt mixture until fully incorporated.

5. Transfer to the lined tin and swirl the remaining mango on top. Fold the clingfilm over the tin and place in the freezer for 4–6 hours or overnight.

6. Remove from the freezer about 30 minutes before you are ready to serve.

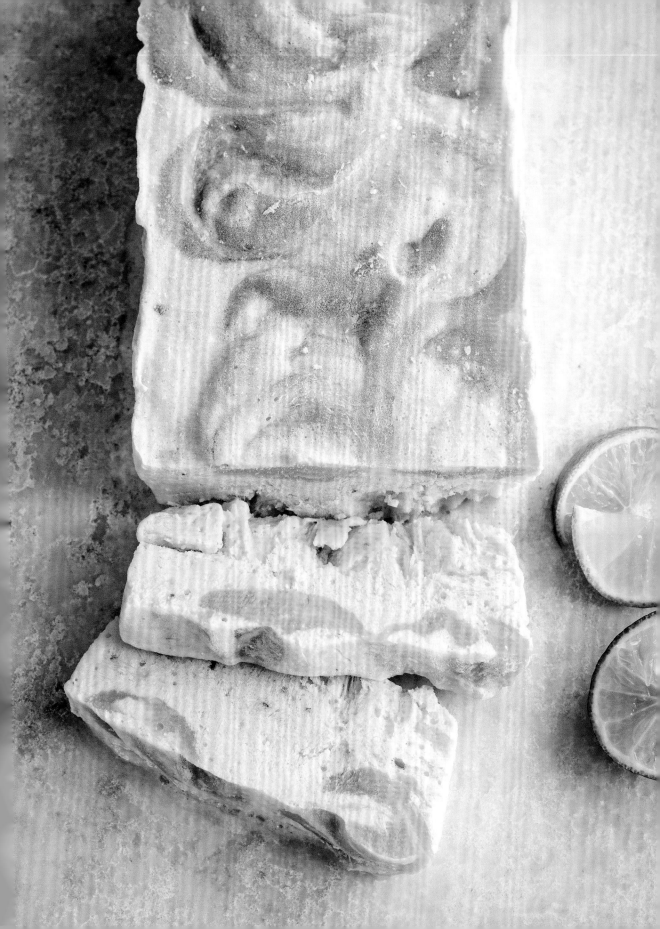

PER SERVING | **95cals** | PROTEIN **7.4g** | CARBS **6.6g**

Vanilla Panna Cotta with Berries

SERVES | PREP
2 | **10–15** mins

1 sheet leaf gelatine
50ml full-fat milk
130g full-fat Greek yoghurt
1 tbsp vanilla extract or paste
½ tsp honey
60g mixed berries, to serve

A mix of Greek yoghurt and milk is used to make these panna cottas ultra silky and light.

1. Place the leaf gelatine in a bowl of water to soften.

2. Heat the milk in a small saucepan until just below boiling point. Remove the pan from the heat. Transfer the softened gelatine to the hot milk and stir until completely dissolved.

3. Mix the yoghurt, vanilla extract or paste and honey together in a medium bowl until smooth. Stir the milk into the yoghurt mixture. Divide between two small glasses and refrigerate for at least 3 hours, until set.

4. To serve, half fill a bowl with hot water. Dip the bases of the glasses into the water and leave for a few seconds. Tip the panna cottas onto a plate and gently tap the bottom of the glass to release. Divide the berries between the two plates and serve.

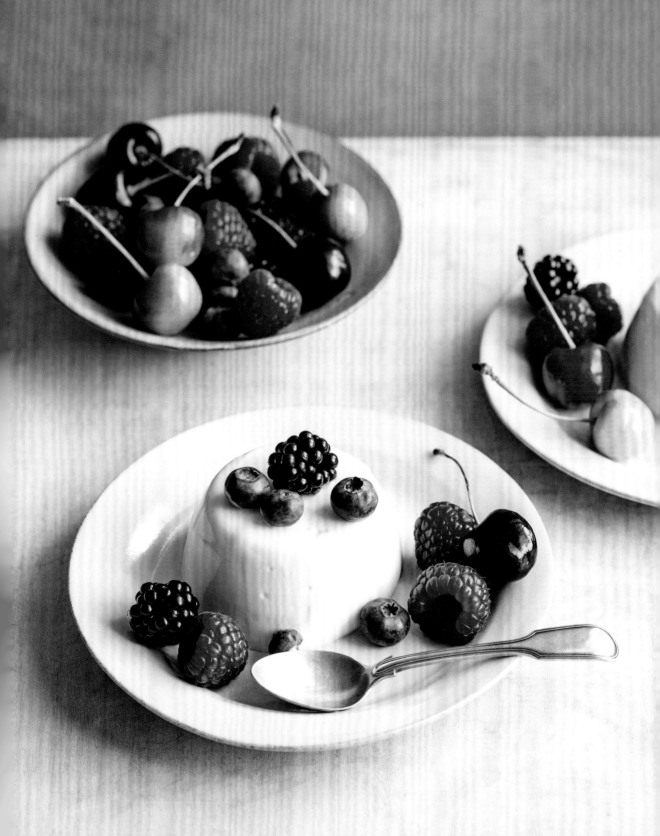

No-count Dressings

PER SERVING | **75cals** | PROTEIN **1.5g** | CARBS **3.2g**

Sriracha Yoghurt Dressing

Sriracha has to be one of our favourite seasonings, adding a burst of sweet chilli and garlic. It's available in most big supermarkets.

SERVES **2** | PREP **2** mins

2 tbsp full-fat Greek yoghurt
1 tbsp full-fat mayonnaise
1½ tbsp sriracha

1. Mix all the ingredients together in a small bowl, jug or jar.

2. The dressing will keep in the fridge for up to a week.

COOK'S TIP

A squeeze of lime juice is a nice addition to this dressing – 1 teaspoon will suffice.

PER SERVING | **125cals** | PROTEIN **0.8g** | CARBS **1.3g**

Miso Dressing

Miso paste (available in a jar) comes from Japan originally. Made of fermented beans, it produces a remarkably versatile, sweet, umami dressing.

SERVES **2** | PREP **2–3** mins

2 tbsp olive oil
1 tbsp white miso paste
1 tbsp cider vinegar
1 tsp sesame oil

1. Whisk all the ingredients together in a small bowl until emulsified. Season with a little freshly ground black pepper.

COOK'S TIP

The dressing will keep well in the fridge.

Curried Yoghurt Dressing

Mildly curry flavoured, this goes with almost anything!

SERVES **2** | PREP **5** mins

2 tbsp full-fat Greek yoghurt
1 tbsp full-fat mayonnaise
1 tsp curry powder
A few stems of coriander, leaves picked
  and finely chopped (optional)

1. Place all the ingredients in a small bowl and mix together. Season to taste with salt and freshly ground black pepper.

French Dressing with Tofu

This is a high-protein take on a classic French dressing. When the ingredients are blended together, it is almost like mayonnaise, but lighter and fluffier. A fabulous dressing to add to your repertoire.

SERVES **2** | PREP **5** mins

2 tbsp olive oil
2 tbsp white wine vinegar
1 tbsp Dijon mustard
2 tbsp silken tofu (approx. 30g)

1. Measure all the ingredients into a jug and use a stick blender to blitz everything together until silky smooth. Season generously with salt and freshly ground black pepper.

2. The dressing will keep in the fridge for up to 5 days.

COOK'S TIP
Excess tofu can be frozen in portions.

Ranch Dressing

Our version of an American classic.

SERVES **2** | PREP **5** mins

2 tbsp full-fat Greek yoghurt
1 tbsp full-fat mayonnaise
½ tsp garlic granules
1 tsp lemon juice
5g fresh flat-leaf parsley,
    finely chopped

1. Mix all the ingredients together
in a small bowl and season with salt
and lots of freshly ground black pepper.

Peanut and Chilli Dressing

A salty, spicy Asian-inspired dressing
with a little sweetness from the peanut
butter. Drizzle it over warm steamed
veg, use in a stir-fry or even as a
dipping sauce.

SERVES **2** | PREP **5** mins

2 tsp smooth unsweetened
    peanut butter
2 tsp sriracha
2 tsp soy sauce

1. Place all the ingredients in a small
bowl and mix together until completely
smooth. Stir in 2 teaspoons of warm
water to loosen, if necessary.

PER SERVING | **79cals** | PROTEIN **0.4g** | CARBS **3.4g**

Asian Dressing

Bring your salad to life with an Asian-inspired dressing – it works well in coleslaws, crunchy salads or drizzled on fish or tofu.

SERVES **2** | PREP **3–4** mins

1 tbsp rapeseed or olive oil
1 tbsp apple cider vinegar
1 tbsp soy sauce
1 tbsp finely grated fresh root ginger
1 tsp sesame oil
½ tsp honey (optional)

1. Place all the ingredients in a small bowl, jug or jar, season with a pinch of salt and a generous grind of black pepper and mix well.

2. The dressing will keep in the fridge for up to a week.

PER SERVING | **108cals** | PROTEIN **0.1g** | CARBS **1.9g**

Balsamic Dressing

A classic, tangy-sweet, dark dressing – one of our family favourites. Having a vinaigrette dressing with a leafy salad improves the absorption of the nutrients in the greens, as well as reducing any potential sugar spike – particularly when eaten at the start of the meal.

SERVES **2** | PREP **5** mins

2 tbsp olive oil
1 tbsp balsamic dressing
½ tsp Dijon mustard
½ tsp dried thyme

1. Place all the ingredients in a small bowl or jug, season with salt and freshly ground black pepper, and whisk together until emulsified.

Protein Top-ups

Maintaining an adequate protein intake is particularly important when you are fasting. We recommend eating a minimum of 50g protein on fast days, and almost double that when you are eating normally on non-fast days – i.e. 70–80g per day for women and 90–100g for men. Protein is needed for the healthy function of all biological systems, including producing hormones, repair and maintaining a healthy immune system. It also makes meals more filling – here are some simple suggestions to help you. Remember, if you want to add a little something, always choose a protein add-on, or some more non-starchy veg, rather than carbohydrate.

Dairy & egg

1 tbsp grated cheese, around 10g
  (41cals, 2.5g protein)
40g Greek yoghurt (53cals, 2g protein)
1 medium boiled egg (78cals, 7g protein)
20g Parmesan, grated (82cals, 7g protein)
30g Cheddar (124cals, 7.5g protein)
50g feta (124cals, 7.5g protein)
30g halloumi, sliced, lightly fried in 1 tsp
  olive oil for 4–5 mins (130cals, 6g protein)
50g soft cheese, such as Brie
  (171cals, 10g protein)
50g soft blue cheese, such as Roquefort,
  (187cals, 10g protein)

Fish

75g frozen cooked prawns, defrosted
  (52cals, 11.5g protein)
45g tuna, canned in oil (72cals, 11.5g protein)
3 drained anchovies in oil (17cals, 2g protein)
1 smoked mackerel fillet, around 70g
  (211cals, 15g protein)
2 slices smoked salmon, around 50g in total
  (92cals, 11.5g protein)
100g roasted or poached salmon
  (239cals, 24.5g protein)

Meat

1 tbsp chopped fried bacon, around 7g
  (24cals, 1.5g protein)
1 tbsp diced chorizo, around 10g
  (40cals, 2.5g protein)
2 thin slices ham, around 40g
  (43cals, 7g protein)
1 rasher cooked back bacon, around 20g
  (61cals, 5g protein)
2 slices roast turkey breast, around 50g
  (76cals, 17g protein)
4 slices salami or cured chorizo, around 20g
  (88cals, 4g protein)
75g cooked chicken breast
  (115cals, 22.5g protein)
2 slices roast beef, around 80g
  (140cals, 26g protein)
Salami Crisps (see page 196)

Vegetarian

40g mushrooms fried in 1 tsp olive oil
  (33cals, 1g protein)
2 tsp sesame seeds, around 10g
  (63cals, 2g protein)
Handful of nuts, around 10g total weight,
  e.g. walnuts, pecans, hazelnuts
  (71cals, 2g protein)
15g flaked almonds (95cals, 4g protein)
100g canned beans (109cals, 7g protein)
80g cooked edamame beans
  (110cals, 9g protein)
2 tbsp mixed seeds, around 20g
  (122cals, 5.4g protein)
100g tofu (123cals, 12.5g protein)
100g cooked lentils (143cals, 11g protein)
100g cooked puy lentils (143cals, 11g protein)
2 tbsp hummus, around 50g
  (160cals, 3.5g protein)
100g cooked quinoa (185cals, 6g protein)
Soy Roasted Seeds (see page 194)
Oven-roasted Spiced Chickpeas (see page 194)

Healthy Complex Carbs

Wholegrains, beans and pulses contain important nutrients and are an excellent source of fibre. They are also a particularly good source of protein for vegetarians. We have included wholegrains in small quantities in some of our recipes. But if you have calories to spare you might add 1 or possibly 2 tablespoons to a dish. On a non-fasting day, you can add 2–3 tablespoons to your meal. Here are a few options:

1 tbsp cooked brown rice (21cals)
1 tbsp cooked quinoa (18cals)
1 tbsp cooked bulgur wheat (13cals)
1 tbsp cooked Puy lentils (18cals)
1 tbsp cooked pearl barley (19cals)

As these foods often take longer to cook, you can save yourself time by cooking larger quantities and freezing them in portions. Try crumbling in half a stock cube during cooking for added flavour.

Other low-carb swaps

Cauli-rice (see page 68)
Courgetti (100g) 20cals
Allow 1 courgette per person (see pages 71 and 72 for ways to cook this)
Green Cauli Mash (see page 182)
Garlicky Mashed Turnips and Cauliflower (see page 182)
Halloumi Fries (see page 196)
Cabbage Pappardelle (see page 74)
Konjak 'Zero' noodles or spaghetti (Shiritaki). Originally from Japan, these contain remarkably few calories and plenty of fibre. They are available in most large supermarkets.

Simple Greens and Non-starchy Veg

Greens and non-starchy vegetables are such an important part of your diet that you should eat them freely without counting the calories. They include: cabbage, spring greens, chard, kale, pak choi, cavolo nero and spinach; as well as fine green beans, mangetout, sliced courgette or broccoli. And salad leaves of all colours – the more colourful, the better the nutritional value (and they look so enticing too).

If it helps you eat them regularly, we encourage you to try these ways to add flavour. Seasoning for a start – flaked sea salt or soy sauce and freshly ground pepper will make a big difference! A pinch of dried chilli flakes, for lovers of heat, or a little crushed garlic are also good, and a squeeze of lemon or lime juice over some broccoli or cabbage goes really well.

Some other low-calorie ways to add flavour:

1 tsp butter (25cals) – good on any veg
1 tsp olive oil (27cals) – good on any veg
1 tsp hoisin sauce (12cals) – try this on wilted spinach or steamed broccoli florets
1 tsp nigella or sesame seeds (32cals) – sprinkle over green beans or cabbage
1 tsp grated Parmesan – scatter on top of roasted courgette or cauliflower florets

Index of Recipes by Calories

UNDER 400 CALORIES

7-DAY MEAL PLANS
2 or 3 Meals a Day, with or without meat

These meal plans are intended to give you a taste of how to mix and match the recipes to make up an 800–900 day. Do feel free to use up your leftovers and swap in different recipes you like the look of or to repeat days, so you don't have to cook two days in a row – whatever best suits you. Just keep an eye on the nutritional information on the recipe pages to make sure you are keeping protein high (more than 50g daily if you can) and starchy carbs and sugar lowish (ideally below 50g).

Remember, the 800–900cals a day is just a ballpark figure. Calories, although useful, are not an accurate science and going over by 40–50cals here and there is not going to make a significant difference to your rate of weight loss. It's the quality of the food that matters. Eating 800cals of pastries (which is surprisingly easy to do!), is going to be far worse for you than 1000cals on a Med-style keto diet.

You will see that in the meat-free plans the daily calorie totals tend to be higher, between 900 and 1000, which is fine. This is to ensure adequate daily protein is included. If you are vegetarian or vegan, you may wish to swap in a suitable high-protein shake to top up your protein (see thefast800.com for options). Equally, on some days, the daily calorie quota falls far enough below the 800cals mark for you to have a treat (see pages 203–35).

You are encouraged on any Fast 800 plan to eat as much leafy and non-starchy veg as you can – you might want to choose a No-count Dressing (see page 236–9) for this or try some of the other ideas on page 240. You can also include a portion of hard fruit, such as an apple or pear, or a handful of berries – to be eaten either with, or straight after, a meal.

The important thing, if you want to encourage fat-burning, is to stick to the portion size in our recipes, avoid snacking between meals, and ideally add in some Time Restricted Eating (see page 11 for more on this).

2 Meals a Day, with Meat

Day 1	Cals / Pro / Carb	Total Cals	Total Pro
Smashed Avocado on Fried Halloumi with Tomatoes and Egg (see page 23)	424 / 23.5 / 3.2		
Chicken Casserole with Chorizo, Thyme and Olives (see page 121)	458 / 43.4 / 17	882	66.9
Day 2			
Harissa Yoghurt with Soft-boiled Eggs and Spinach (see page 24)	228 / 20.6 / 2.1		
Chargrilled Rib-eye Steak with Romesco and Broccoli (see page 146)	594 / 57.1 / 5.9	822	77.7
Day 3			
Warm Crispy Kale Salad with Mushrooms, Bacon and Goat's Cheese (see page 56)	285 / 13.4 / 1.3		
Keto-fried Chicken (see page 112)	555 / 55.4 / 2.6	840	68.8
Day 4			
Cottage Cheese Crepes with Bacon, Avocado and Oven-roasted Tomatoes (see page 30)	365 / 16.1 / 9.8		
Duck Breasts with Rocket, Mustard and Puy Lentils (see page 129)	509 / 55.4 / 15.4	874	71.5
Day 5			
Courgetti with Prawns and Creamy Garlic Sauce (see page 71)	380 / 28 / 4		
Baked Pork with Winter Vegetables (see page 142)	420 / 48.7 / 12.6	800	76.7
Day 6			
Cauli-rice Kedgeree (see page 40)	473 / 40.3 / 27.4		
One Pan Squeezed Sausage Casserole (see page 140)	525 / 22.7 / 15.2	998	63
Day 7			
Spiced Baked Beans with Cavolo Nero and Egg (see page 178)	286 / 14.8 / 19.2		
Piri Piri Roast Chicken with Jalapeno Yoghurt (see page 116)	377 / 56.9 / 4.4		
With Green Cauli Mash (see page 182)	102 / 4.1 / 5.3		
And Vanilla Panna Cotta with Berries (see page 234)	95 / 7.4 / 6.6	860	83.2

3 Meals a Day, with Meat

Day 1	Cals / Pro / Carb	Total Cals	Total Pro
Cauli-rice Kedgeree (see page 40)	473 / 40.3 / 27.4		
Creamy Broccoli, Ginger and Coriander Soup (see page 52)	293 / 5.1 / 6.9		
Baked Tandoori Chicken with Garlic Raita (see page 114)	210 / 27.4 / 3.9	**976**	**72.8**

Day 2			
Blueberry Bircher Muesli (see page 20)	209 / 6.8 / 18.1		
Thai Pork Lettuce Cups (see page 78)	274 / 24.8 / 3.4		
Bang Bang Chicken (see page 122)	377 / 44 / 8	**860**	**75.6**

Day 3			
Mushroom and Miso Eggs with Spinach (see page 28)	195 / 16.8 / 1.4		
With Cloud Bread (see page 205)	56 / 4 / 0.3		
Chicken and Egg Noodle Soup (see page 48)	253 / 38.3 / 0.5		
Greek Turkey Burgers with Harissa Yoghurt (see page 132)	327 / 34.9 / 6.3	**831**	**94**

Day 4			
Keto Granola Breakfast Bowl (see page 22)	232 / 10.8 / 7.1		
Pesto Courgetti Spaghetti with Red Pepper and Feta (see page 72)	331 / 12.5 / 6.6		
Easy Lamb Koftas with Green Salad and Harissa Yoghurt (see page 153)	320 / 28 / 5.4	**800**	**51.3**

Day 5			
Blueberry and Chocolate Protein Smoothie (see page 20)	251 / 17.6 / 22.9		
Sriracha Prawn Cocktail Protein Wrap (see page 66)	253 / 18.9 / 6.6		
Easy Sausage Traybake with White Beans (see page 143)	364 / 20.5 / 26	**868**	**57**

Day 6			
Baked Eggs in Peppers (see page 33)	242 / 16.2 / 3.2		
Chicken Liver Pâté (see page 76)	213 / 7.9 / 3.7		
Spicy Salmon and Butternut Squash Traybake (see page 100)	512 / 31.1 / 17.4	**967**	**55.2**

Day 7			
Cottage Cheese Crepes with Bacon, Avocado and Oven-roasted Tomatoes (see page 30)	365 / 16.1 / 9.8		
Cajun Cauliflower Soup with Silken Tofu (see page 51)	132 / 6.7 / 7.1		
Tandoori Lamb Cutlets with Garlic and Ginger Spinach (see page 154)	415 / 38.9 / 6.8	**912**	**61.7**

2 Meals a Day, Vegetarian

Day 1	Cals / Pro / Carb	Total Cals	Total Pro
Smashed Avocado on Fried Halloumi with Tomatoes and Egg (see page 23)	424 / 23.5 / 3.2		
Pink Cauli Risotto with Halloumi and Spinach (see page 68)	427 / 24.4 / 16.6		
With Mocha Mousse Pots with Strawberries (see page 227)	123 / 6 / 11.2	**974**	**53.9**

Day 2			
Harissa Yoghurt with Soft-boiled Eggs and Spinach (see page 24)	228 / 20.6 / 2.1		
With Soy Roasted Seeds (see page 194)	77 / 3.3 / 2.3		
Warm Orange and Walnut Salad with Halloumi (see page 160)	449 / 19.4 / 7.6		
With Instant Mug Bread (see page 206)	245 / 9.6 / 2.7	**999**	**52.3**

Day 3			
Veg and Egg Breakfast Bake (see page 26)	276 / 21.8 / 6.2		
With Cloud Bread (see page 205)	56 / 4 / 0.3		
Glazed Ginger and Garlic Tofu with Spinach (see page 177)	308 / 19 / 4.6		
With Persian Love Cake (see page 209)	273 / 8 / 9.8	**913**	**52.8**

Day 4			
Scrambled Eggs with Harissa Sautéed Kale and Soy Roasted Seeds (see page 38)	249 / 20.1 / 2.9		
With Instant Mug Bread (see page 206)	245 / 9.6 / 2.7		
Cauli Cheese with Jalapeño Peppers (see page 171)	467 / 20.5 / 13.7	**961**	**50.2**

Day 5			
Pink Cauli Risotto with Halloumi and Spinach (see page 68)	427 / 24.4 / 16.6		
Teriyaki Tofu Stir-fry (see page 176)	440 / 23.7 / 15.8		
With Instant Rhubarb Pudding with Diced Stem Ginger (see page 224)	257 / 8.9 / 11.9	**1124**	**57**

Day 6			
Spiced Baked Beans with Cavolo Nero and Egg (see page 178)	286 / 14.8 / 19.2		
With Instant Mug Bread (see page 206)	245 / 9.6 / 2.7		
Glazed Ginger and Garlic Tofu with Spinach (see page 177)	308 / 19 / 4.6		
With Persian Love Cake (see page 209)	273 / 8 / 9.8	**1112**	**51.4**

Day 7			
Teriyaki Tofu Stir-fry (see page 176)	440 / 23.7 / 15.8		
With Chocolate Peanut Butter Cookie (see page 217)	58 / 2.3 / 4.2		
Roasted Pepper and Halloumi Eggs (see page 29)	324 / 22.3 / 5.9		
With Oven-roasted Spiced Chickpeas (see page 194)	109 / 4.8 / 10	**931**	**53.1**

3 Meals a Day, Vegetarian

Day 1	Cals / Pro / Carb	Total Cals	Total Pro
Mushroom and Miso Eggs with Spinach (see page 28)	195 / 16.8 / 1.4		
Warm Orange and Walnut Salad with Halloumi (see page 160)	449 / 19.4 / 7.6		
Roasted Veg with Feta, Almonds and Red Pepper Sauce (see page 166)	457 / 17.9 / 14	**1101**	**54.1**
Day 2			
Scrambled Eggs with Harissa Sautéed Kale and Soy Roasted Seeds (see page 38)	249 / 20.1 / 2.9		
Creamy Egg Salad (see page 61)	214 / 15.2 / 2.7		
With Instant Mug Bread (see page 206)	245 / 9.6 / 2.7		
French Bean Bowl with Feta and Pine Nuts (see page 165)	328 / 12.7 / 7.6	**1036**	**57.6**
Day 3			
Greek Scrambled Eggs (see page 37)	276 / 15.3 / 3.5		
With Cloud Bread (see page 205)	56 / 4 / 0.3		
Pesto Courgetti Spaghetti with Red Pepper and Feta (see page 72)	331 / 12.5 / 6.6		
Egg-fried Cauli and Broccoli Rice (see page 175)	258 / 14.3 / 15.8		
With Vanilla Panna Cotta with Berries (see page 234)	95 / 7.4 / 6.6	**1016**	**53.5**
Day 4			
Roasted Pepper and Halloumi Eggs (see page 29)	324 / 22.3 / 5.9		
Cajun Cauliflower Soup with Silken Tofu (see page 51)	132 / 6.7 / 7.1		
Green Vegetable Gratin (see page 163)	422 / 13.9 / 5.6		
With Chocolate and Fruit Chia Yoghurt Pot (see page 231)	182 / 9.4 / 13.8	**1060**	**52.3**
Day 5			
Blueberry and Chocolate Protein Smoothie (see page 20)	251 / 17.6 / 22.9		
Easy Garlicky Mushrooms (see page 159)	266 / 13.1 / 1.5		
Halloumi Skewers with Coleslaw (see page 172)	322 / 16.8 / 9.8		
With Mocha Mousse Pots with Strawberries (see page 227)	123 / 6 / 11.2	**962**	**53.5**
Day 6			
Keto Granola Breakfast Bowl (see page 22)	232 / 10.8 / 7.1		
Black Bean and Mango Slaw (see page 54)	332 / 11.3 / 27.5		
With Oven-roasted Spiced Chickpeas (see page 194)	109 / 4.8 / 10		
Teriyaki Tofu Stir-fry (see page 176)	440 / 23.7 / 15.8	**1113**	**50.6**
Day 7			
Black Olive and Toasted Almond Eggs (see page 29)	352 / 16.8 / 7.3		
Pear and Rosemary Muffin (see page 210)	160 / 7.1 / 4.1		
Pink Cauli Risotto with Halloumi and Spinach (see page 68)	427 / 24.4 / 16.6		
With Chocolate Florentine (see page 212)	112 / 2.2 / 8.8	**1051**	**50.5**

Index

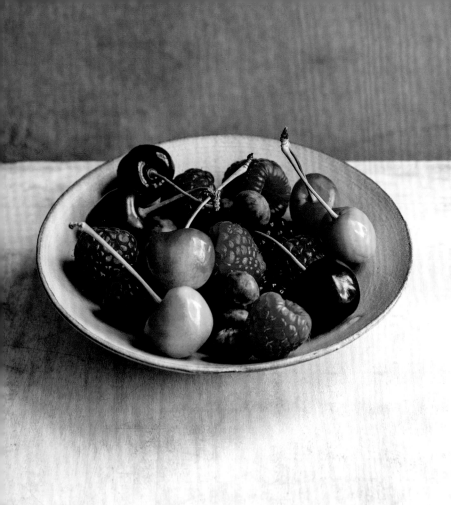

DR CLARE BAILEY, wife of Michael Mosley, has supported hundreds of patients during her medical career to lose weight, reduce their blood sugars and put their diabetes into remission. She is the author of the bestselling *8-Week Blood Sugar Diet Recipe Book*, *Clever Guts Diet Recipe Book*, *Fast 800 Recipe Book* and *The Fast 800 Easy*.

Instagram @drclarebailey

KATHRYN BRUTON is a recipe writer, developer and food stylist who contributes to the UK's bestselling cookbooks and leading food magazines. She is the author of her own bestselling series of low-calorie, high-nutrition cookbooks and now collaborates with leading authors to curate dynamic, must-cook recipes.

Instagram @kathryn_bruton